LISA A. SHATFORD
DEPARTMENT OF PSYCHOLOGY
UNIVERSITY HOSPITAL
P.O. BOX 5339, STN. A.
LONDON, ONTARIO   N6A 5A5
CANADA   (519) 663-3461

GIVE US A CHILD

Coping with
the Personal Crisis
of Infertility

Lynda Rutledge Stephenson

1817

Harper & Row, Publishers, San Francisco

Cambridge, Hagerstown, New York, Philadelphia, Washington
London, Mexico City, São Paulo, Singapore, Sydney

Grateful acknowledgment is made for use from "Yours, Mine and Theirs," by Lori B. Andrews, *Psychology Today*, Dec. 1984. Copyright 1984 by *Psychology Today*. Reprinted by permission.

FIRST EDITION

Library of Congress Cataloging-in-Publication Data

Stephenson, Lynda Rutledge.
  Give us a child.

  Bibliography: p.
  Includes index.
  1. Infertility—Religious aspects—Christianity.
  2. Infertility—Psychological aspects.   I. Title.
  RC889.S726   1987   248.8'6   86-45830
  ISBN 0-06-067591-8

---

87 88 89 90 91 HC 10 9 8 7 6 5 4 3 2 1

ACKNOWLEDGMENTS

Some special people:
Suzii Paynter
Jim and Elaine Karban
Jose Pliego, M.D.
Marge Vogt, R.N.
Robert Grayson, M.D.
Jeanne Fleming, Ph.D.
Patricia Mahlstedt, Ed.D.
Beverly Freeman, RESOLVE
Merle Bombardieri, MSW
    and especially, Roy M. Carlisle of Harper & Row
    San Francisco

Whether through information or guidance,
through sharing or brainstorming,
through moral support or friendship,
you've helped me through this experience
better than you know.

Thanks with all my heart.

To Don

CONTENTS

PROLOGUE

Good for you.

You've taken the first positive step toward dealing with what may—or may not—become a major life crisis. You just don't know, and not knowing is rough. You're beginning to wonder whether maybe, just maybe there might be a problem. You may not have confided your fears to anyone yet. You may not even have talked with your doctor yet. Or you may be well into the merry-go-round of tests. But you have decided you need to know what is going on and, more importantly, how to handle it. And that is a very, very big step—a step that many never have the courage to take.

Don't let anyone tell you that infertility isn't a major life crisis. It is. Friends, family, and acquaintances may shrug it off with casual remarks like:

"Just relax," or

"You're lucky. Kids are a pain," or

"Pull yourself together. It's not like you have cancer or anything," or, even,

"Hey, don't worry about it. You two will get the hang of it soon. (wink, wink)"

Between you and me, we could probably fill a book with such innocently insensitive remarks. But infertility's quietness, its ambivalent sort of public image doesn't lessen its intensely personal nature or its potentially devastating effects on those involved. Infertility is a major life crisis, all right, and it should be treated as such.

This may sound trite, and it may be of little comfort, but,

believe me, I know what you're going through. Everything you're going through. I know the denial that has kept you from facing the question mark on your plans for the future. I know the monthly depression of being unable to deny it. I know the unaskable questions that are continually surfacing in your mind, questions that can jolt the foundations of your marriage, your self-image, your beliefs.

The book that you hold in your hands is a product of my need to know, my need to cope . . . as infertility took every one of my bedrock beliefs about myself and my life and flipped them upside down. When my husband and I began trudging through the infertility process, I found very little information that met our needs in the personal areas of emotions and ethics and faith. And what I did find left me wanting and needing more.

Very normally, my husband and I wanted infertility to be like other medical problems. We wanted the doctor to give us a pill that would make everything all right. But infertility isn't like other medical problems—we came to understand that all too quickly. How many medical problems involve two people? How many are loaded with social reverberations? How many may force you to face your own ethics? Or challenge your faith?

How were we supposed to juggle all these very different issues as we lived with our desire to have a child? We needed answers. And so began our search. Or more correctly—the search was forced upon us . . . as it has been upon you.

This book was written to help you in that search, to help you gain perspective on this touchy, intimate, personal dilemma. It isn't exactly easy to read. It wasn't easy to write. But the writing of it has taught me much.

I hope the reading of it does the same for you.

"Well, how'd it go?"

I hop into the car as my husband pulls out of the doctor's parking lot and into traffic. "Well?" *he persists.* "What'd he say?"

"Oh, lots of things. It went pretty well. Says he's gonna get us pregnant. No problem."

"No problem, huh."

"That's what he said," *I answer with a slight grin. I wave a piece of paper in front of his nose.* "Got a minute? We need to go by the drugstore—make it the supermarket. They've got a pharmacy."

"What are we buying?" *my husband asks.*

"A thermometer. A 'B-a-s-a-l' thermometer," *I read from the paper in my hand.*

"A what?" *he asks, one eyebrow cocked.*

"Don't worry. You *don't* have to use it. It's for me."

"Good."

"Yeah, I thought you'd like that," *I mutter, looking out of the corner of my eye at him.* "Something about timing ovulation. I think my temperature dips when I'm ovulating. Or does it rise? Something like that," *I mumble as I look back down at the paper.* Sounds simple enough, *I think.* Then again, I thought getting pregnant was simple.

We ride in silence for a moment. He drives. I watch the cars passing by. A blue VW. One of those little pick-ups, Datsun maybe. A Chrysler station wagon with three kids, and a dog—ears flapping in the wind. Had it really been two years since we had decided to start a family? We'd gotten all our education, all our misgivings, all our settling in—out of the way. And we'd made the big decision.

Then nothing. We turned thirty. Still nothing. Maybe we had waited too long. Maybe we were trying too hard.

"Wanna go to a movie tonight?" my husband asks, laying his hand over mine.

I shrug.

"Okay, how about a movie and dinner?"

"Fast food or real food?"

"You drive a hard bargain . . . real." He drives up in front of the supermarket's door. *"I'll be back in a few minutes to pick you up and we'll decide."* I jump out of the car and walk around to his side. *"It's gonna help,"* he says, leaning out of the car window. *"Don't worry."*

"I know," I smile, then turn and walk through the electronic door.

Inside, I grab a cart and almost bump into a very pregnant woman beside me.

"Whoops!" she says. *"ExCUSE me! Kinda hard to miss me at this point, haha."*

"Haha," I echo, then steer around her and down the first aisle.

Baby foods, baby bibs, baby rattlers, industrial size boxes of Pampers surround me. Dozens of pictures of happy babies smile down from the shelves. Unable to help myself, I smile back. I pick up a little three-sectioned yellow dish decorated with a cute cartoon bear's face; it rattles happily from somewhere underneath. Strangely enough, I start to set it in my cart. Then I stop, and, shaking my head, silently laugh at myself. Positive thinking, Lynda? I think, as I set it back on the shelf.

"Well, what brand do you recommend?" I hear ahead of me, and look up to see two pregnant women standing in front of the strained green beans. They are talking of swollen ankles and baby formula and due dates as I stroll past and turn down the next aisle: toys, sporting goods, games. A small boy looks up at me as he takes a toy car for a test drive. His pregnant mother comes from out of nowhere and carts him away.

"Good grief," I mumble. *"Is this pregnant day at the supermarket?"* Or . . . am I going to start noticing every pregnant woman on earth? *I finger my prescription nervously and head toward the drug counter. And for the briefest moment I am agitated at my fertile friends and their effortless conceptions, and at the whole normal world who only buy normal thermometers for normal reasons.*

"Hi, can I help you?" the young male clerk asks.

"I hope so," I say quietly, handing him the piece of paper. "Boy, I certainly hope so. . . ."

INTRODUCTION

"So, when are you two gonna have a baby?"

Sound familiar? Sometimes it seems as if the whole world is asking that personal question. Well . . . maybe it is. There's no debating that the world is quite busy being fruitful and multiplying, and that it views doing so as natural and expected. And those who aren't, well, they will be sooner or later. It's all a matter of choice, after all. No problem.

But . . . there *can* be a problem. And when it strikes home, the problem can easily slide right into a major life crisis, one that multiplies into a series of crises: a medical crisis, for sure—but just as profoundly, a social one, an emotional and psychological one, a marital one, and for many, an ethical and spiritual one.

The *medical crisis* is the most visible one. Because the other issues either coincide with it or are fueled by it, the medical experience is usually the hub of the whole infertility crisis. It begins when you finally voice that sneaking suspicion floating around in the back of your mind, make that first doctor's appointment, and begin the infertility medical work-up. And then you begin learning words such as "post-coital," and "basal body thermometer," and "hysterosalpingogram"; you find yourself on a first name basis with the nurse who takes your blood tests; and "infertility" becomes a household word.

Infertility—it's an awful sounding medical term, one that never loses its tinny sound or its bitter taste. But it's not a hopeless word, by any means. And although taking that step into the doctor's office seems ominous and loaded with unpleasant things such as pills and tests and treatments, it *can* be a momentous and hopeful step. For the majority of couples, it is the first step toward the solution.

But the trauma of the medical work-up is just one part of the infertility experience. The social crisis of infertility is inescapable, because even though infertility is an intensely personal matter, your very private business becomes a very public matter. Grandma's hinting. Aunt Fanny's wondering. Your friends are waxing poetic about LaMaze and baby food. People you hardly know flash pictures of their family's latest addition in front of you. And there you are.

The pressure is bad enough for the couple who has chosen to be childless, but for the couple who wants a child desperately, who has been trying for years, who may be riding the infertility roller coaster of tests and pills and doctors, every insensitive remark is an arrow—aimed dead center for the heart.

So, it becomes easier not to go to that family reunion or annual picnic than to hear: "Hi, nice to meet you. How many children do you have?" or "You two aren't getting any younger, you know. . . ." or "Here, want to hold the baby?" And it's easier not to get together with your friends when Little League is what's happening in their lives and temperature charting is what's happening in yours.

Every diaper commercial, every baby shower, every Christmas and Mother's Day only remind you of what you don't have. And every bit of well-meaning advice ("Eat oysters." "Take vitamin E." "Stand on your head afterwards." "Start jogging." "Quit jogging.") makes a very natural, joyful part of married life seem like mission impossible. You begin to isolate yourself, feel alone, feel that life is at a standstill. And you suddenly become aware of your biological clock ticking, ticking, ticking. . . .

Yet, believe it or not, you are not alone. In fact, the latest figures state that nearly one out of every five couples in America today has trouble with infertility. *One out of every five.*[1] *Newsweek* is telling us so. Publications as varied as *Time, Reader's Digest, Glamour, Business Week, Science News, Better Homes & Gardens,* and *American Health* (to name only a very few) have given—and continue to give—time and space to the topic of infertility. It's that timely. Even syndicated columnists Ann Landers and Erma Bombeck have written about this growing, modern phenomenon you are experiencing. The number of couples coping with some sort of infertility has doubled in the last fifteen years. And society is finally waking up to this fact of modern life. What is happening?

For the first time ever, a generation of women, my generation, could choose to wait for parenthood. The birth control pill gave us this choice. We could wait and ponder the when's and why's of having a child.

And I did. In my long-range plan, I would surely be a mother. But later—when we both had our education, when we were both more mature. When we weren't so dirt poor. And thousands of others made the same plans. But when later came, a lot of us were in for a shock. It became time to choose motherhood, we chose it . . . and nothing happened.

And nothing happening is happening more and more. Part of the phenomenon can be traced to the obvious fact that a whole generation of women waited until thirty or so to have children. And as we grow older, our fertility diminishes—a fact that very few of us were aware of at the time. Mentally, we can choose to wait; physically, we may not have that choice.

Other factors of modern life come into play, too. We are offered alternatives, but the alternatives may have their lasting conditions. The birth control pill itself may cause a lingering effect, usually temporary, on a woman's ovulation. The IUD

(Intrauterine Device), a very popular form of birth control, causes infection problems for a small percentage of its users, especially those who've never had children. Venereal disease is on the rise. And abortion can have its long-lasting infection hazard. Supposedly, there's also a marked decrease in sperm count among men of all ages, a mystifying situation that researchers suspect might be caused by environmental pollution.[2] There are even medical problems that drugs from a generation ago have caused—as in the case of DES daughters who are prone to miscarry and maybe even to cancer due to the drug DES (Diethystibestrol) their mothers were given so *they* wouldn't miscarry.[3]

But the most elusive factor is panic. We can't help but worry that we might be inhibiting our own fertility just by being overly anxious. Make no mistake, though; most of the time a problem is found. Anxiety just seems to make things worse. Modern medicine is only now beginning to understand the overall effects of stress on the entire body, even though doctors are really not in agreement on what extent such stress is a factor in infertility. The fact, though, that the effects of stress do exist often results in such oversimplistic advice as "Just relax," which even doctors are guilty of saying—and which couples battling infertility are bored to tears of hearing.

Less than twenty years ago, most couples facing some sort of infertility would have had no choice but to accept the situation. Today, we are faced with a myriad of innovative ways to combat infertility, and as we consider them the medical side of the infertility crisis begins.

Then, slowly, almost imperceptibly, the personal and psychological dimensions of the social crisis begin to intrude. And the questions begin:

"How will this affect how others treat us?"

"What will our family say?"

"How will this affect our marriage? Our picture of the future? Our own well-being?"

"*Why* is this happening?"

The stress of infertility can play funny tricks on your mind. It's filled with all sorts of tiny time bombs. Psychologically, you are probably questioning the very basic picture you have had of yourselves and your life as a couple—a family. Psychology has always rated parenting as a developmental level of growth, intimating with its silence that maybe those without children are missing a basic maturity step. Only recently has this been questioned.[4] Can two healthy people be well-balanced, vital, mature adults without children? Who is right? The people who tell us we're lucky or the people who extend sympathy and advice?

Perspective can get all out of whack. Having a baby can become sort of a "holy grail," an all-consuming passion that burns up all other life aspirations——and maybe even your life's most intimate relationship, your marriage. This little time bomb is quite subtle. As you begin grappling with the possibilities of infertility, it doesn't seem so important. But with the stress of wondering what will happen, what the problem is, and even whose problem it is, you'll begin to wonder: Is the effort worth the strain it will put my marriage through?

Infertility either pulls a couple together or pulls them apart. It very rarely leaves the marriage untouched. The awkwardness of discussing the intimate details of your sexual relationship with a doctor and the routine of tests and schedules is bad enough. But with the tyranny of temperature charts and timed lovemaking, it's very easy to feel as if there are three people in your bedroom at night: you, your husband, and your doctor. Even the best of marriages will feel the pressure, especially if one of you falls into the trap of becoming obsessed with having what you fear you may not ever have—to the exclusion of everything and everyone around you. Those feelings, left unattended, unfaced and undiscussed, are emotional plutonium.

And that's when you suddenly realize the breadth of infertility's emotional impact. The couple facing a fertility problem will be dragged, dazed and numb, through countless emotions—fear, shock, distress, hope, depression, grief, sadness, loneliness, anger—you name it, you'll feel it. And it seems that every one of them sneaks up on you unexpectedly.

Sometimes you'll experience them together, you and your spouse. But often, most often, you're on your emotional own. You, the wife, may feel a sudden flash of anger at the woman yelling at a child in the supermarket, or burst into tears as you stroll by a rack of birth announcement cards. And you, the husband, may feel a tinge of envy as your co-worker leaves to attend his son's soccer game, or feel a sense of ambivalence or even annoyance on *the* night of your wife's temperature cycle. Life lived with the ongoing feeling of grief that infertility can produce does more than disrupt dreams, it changes personalities, twisting the very fibers of life. You feel out of control and helpless to change how you feel.

Much of the emotional strain comes straight from unspoken cultural pressures. Certain ideas about our "natural" male and female roles follow us around and echo in our beings: A *real* woman experiences motherhood. . . . A *real* man must have an heir, must prove his masculinity by creating offspring. Wherever they come from, such ancient ideas of fertility and sexuality die hard, and hurt deeply.

Then there's the spiritual crisis. Doesn't the couple with deep personal faith find it easier to cope with this major life crisis? Well, yes and no. In a very real sense, faith can complicate the issue. We believe our faith will be a comfort to us in a crisis, and for many, even those who search and ask questions, it remains so—or ultimately will be so. But the bald fact is that infertility may be worse for the person of religious faith. How? A person who believes that a random fate controls life will suffer the same anxiety, the same grief, the same heartbreak, but if that person blames anything, he or she will blame a faceless, powerless fate.

But who does the person of faith blame? Who do we go to if we're angry with God? Do we store our frustration and our questions, worrying about lightning bolts? Do we attempt a saint's supply of acceptance? Or do we confront them and possibly, just possibly, risk our faith? This is a very real tension for millions of couples who devoutly believe in a God who is involved in the very intimate aspects of daily life. And who want to continue to believe.

And if all these weren't enough, there is the ethical quandary attached to the amazing new biotechnology. And the issue will only become bigger as modern medicine finds more and more alternatives for us to consider. Why? Because we are caught in the middle of a topic that couldn't be more timely. Test-tube fertilization, sperm banks, artificial insemination, surrogate mothers, embryo transfers, genetic engineering . . . words that were found only in science fiction novels a few short years ago are not only possibilities today, but some have become normal procedures. Which of the new procedures are okay? Which are playing God? Which can we consider trying in good conscience? And which should we question? Is this test-tube fertilization really as controversial as it sounds? And what about artificial insemination by donor? With abortion's effect on the number of babies available for adoption, could that be a new way to . . . adopt?

How does a person with strong ethical convictions choose? The decisions won't be easy. Right now, society is attempting to cope with the areas where technology has outstripped our legal system. So for some couples the question will be: What is legal? Others will ask: What do we feel is ethically and morally okay? For some it will be: How does my faith fit into all this? Since most of the new alternatives are laced with religious debate and concern, the ethical question will pose a frustrating, mind-boggling situation for the couple who devoutly believes, who wants to do the right thing—but who also wants to have a baby. The issue is enough to make anyone dizzy, even if you weren't personally involved. But you are. And in essence, "What price a baby?" is the question you may be forced to consider.

Infertility is anything but simple, and more and more of us are finding ourselves in its dilemma, experiencing first hand the problems its tiny time bombs create.

To diffuse as many of these little bombs as possible is the goal of this book. This is a book about the whole experience of infertility, though, and not a medical book per se. So the medical section (Section 3) offers you only a brief overview, created essentially to familiarize you with the important medical aspects of infertility—what infertility is, what causes it, how to pick a specialist, what to expect from your basic medical work-up, what the new procedures are. The section's purpose will be to give you the kind of information you need to begin your medical trek and then to point you toward learning more.

Why should you learn more? Doctors, however caring and patient they may be, cannot teach you all there is to know or fulfill your *need* to know, as it should be filled. I came to that conclusion only after many hours of waiting rooms and examinations. To a doctor, a "hysterosalpingogram" is just a familiar test. To you it's a frightening word and an experience that some knowledge would help you get through. And any doctor worth his diplomas would welcome an informed patient asking informed questions. After all, it's your body.

The medical horizon on infertility is expanding all the time, and so is the literature on it. I urge you to consult some of the excellent books that deal specifically with this aspect of the crisis.

The other crises of infertility, though, are the heart of this book, and are essentially the book's "reason-to-be." The book's order is based on how each one seeped into my own life and awareness—the emotional, the social, and the medical ones somewhat entangled, followed by the ethical and spiritual issues that surfaced as my husband and I were plunged deeper into the matter. The experience may be different for you. So I invite you to read the sections in whatever order they meet your needs, because that's exactly what they're meant to do.

"There they are," my husband says, pointing as he pulls into a parking space at the mall.

Yep, I think, laughing to myself, there they are. What a picture. My sister and her family are waving at us from in front of the mall's entrance. The perfect portrait of the All-American family: husband gently bouncing a toddler in his arms, wife grinning broadly, preteen girl trying to look detached, and young boy squirming and wiggling then wriggling free.

Before I can effectively get out of the car, my five-year-old nephew has bounded over to greet us. He grabs my hand and, as we walk toward the others, bombards me with all the things going on in his little life—important things like getting a stitch in his big toe, and how their new German Shepherd puppy had sat on his chest.

I glance ahead at the mall with its pane after pane of glass in front of us. All the reflections of people coming and going and coming. I notice one reflection: a mother, thirty-ish, holding the hand of her young son. . . .

And suddenly, I realize . . . That's no mother! That's ME! Me and my nephew! My stomach suddenly is in my throat. My nephew is still talking, yet I look away. And I let go of his hand. I realize I'm out of control. Waves of emotion, one after the other, roll over me— eerieness, sadness, frustration, anger . . . even embarrassment, for some crazy reason! As if I had no right to the story that reflection seemed to be telling.

My emotions! I can't stand being so out of control. But it's hap- pening more and more lately. I never know what I'm going to feel or how I'm going to react. One moment, sane, well-adjusted woman. The next—who knows? WHAT is happening to me?! I want to scream. This whole infertility thing is beginning to have a strangle-hold on my feelings, and it is driving me CRAZY! I mean, shouldn't a fairly intelligent woman be able to handle getting a shower invitation or watching a sad movie or—walking into a mall—without going to pieces?

Zipping through my mind are other times I've had this same awful, out-of-control feeling:

- *Last Mother's Day when a grocery cashier asked me what my kids had gotten me . . .* emptiness.
- *At the party I threw where a couple brought their newborn and everyone tried to ignore the tension . . .* embarrassment.
- *At the swimming pool, where I had to stop in mid-lap because I found myself crying . . .* depression.
- *At lunch with my friends listening to talk about soccer and PTA and summer camp and family outings . . .* loneliness.

I fight back the tears. No one knows. We greet the others and walk into the mall. My husband is telling a joke and everyone is laughing. And I am once again in control. Once again.

My nephew is walking quietly a step away. I sigh very quietly, then poke him. He grins. And reaches out for my hand again.

WHY DO I FEEL SO OUT OF CONTROL?

The Emotional Crisis

Out-of-control. That's an adjective no one wants to be labeled with. But the crisis of infertility *is* a crisis of control—you no longer feel you are in control of your future, your plans, your dreams, even your relationships. And the first sign of your inner realization of that loss is the crazy zig-zag path your emotions carry you down. Why else would a normal, basically well-balanced person like you

- skip church on Mother's Day or Father's Day?
- cry when you hear your sister is having her third baby?
- contemplate giving your spouse a divorce so he/she can have children with someone else?
- feel like slapping the pregnant woman riding next to you on the plane?
- become depressed when a test comes back saying you are normal and healthy?
- retreat into your office when your co-workers are celebrating the birth of a friend's new baby?
- wonder if your spouse will still love you if your tubes are scarred or your semen analysis is poor?

- angrily switch the television station when a baby shampoo commercial appears or a happy family sit-com begins?
- keep your infertility a secret as if you've done something wrong?

They sound pretty crazy when you see them in print, don't they? But all of us have done one or all of the above as we've taken those precarious steps into an infertility medical work-up. Yet, we aren't crazy. We're just reacting to a very unusual, doubly stressful crisis in our lives—one that is not easily re-solved, because it is truly not like any other sort of crisis we humans go through. In her book, *New Conceptions*, Lori An-drews explains it this way:

> Infertility touches all aspects of a couple's life. It climbs into bed with them. It colors how they talk to their parents. It dictates their social schedule—arranging vacation plans so that treatment schedules will not be disrupted, and keeping them from showers or christening, where their sadness is overwhelming.

Or as Lynn Drew, a mother after seven years of infertility, put it: "Sex is timed; vacation is timed. It takes a toll in mar-riage, job, body image, everything. It touches every area of our life. Nothing goes unscathed. Nothing."[1]

Why is this crisis so different? Our society doesn't know what to do with us, how to react to us. And so we don't know how to react to it. As Barbara Menning, founder of RESOLVE—the national non-profit infertility organization—explains, "Even in this day of sexual candor, infertility is a difficult sub-ject for many to discuss. It is personal and inherently sexual."[2] Yet in one way or another society intrudes into this personal domain, demanding answers and expecting roles to be filled. It has fashioned our way of thinking, and we cannot help but feel out of step with the whole world.

The pressure is different for women than for men, as are the reactions. Women feel the pressure socially and physically. Be-sides experiencing the bulk of the testing, the wife will face the bulk of the questioning, and most of the "blame." But the most painful pressure may come from within herself, because she may not be fitting into her own personal self-portrait. Where do we get these portraits of our future selves? From our culture. As girls, we were conditioned for the role of mother above every other role in life, while boys were trained to fit into a variety of future roles. Those are our traditional roots. And that's why even though a woman today can be successful in every other area of life, if she isn't a mother, she may feel "unfulfilled."

Men feel the societal pressure sexually. One man explained, "When it was my wife's problem, I could be wonderfully supportive. But when I learned that I had a problem as well, my masculinity was threatened. I resisted surgery for months, provoking our first major marriage conflict."[3]

And men may have good reason to react so strongly. When women finally do open up to their friends, they can receive comfort and support. But it may not be so for a man, due to our culture's preoccupation with sex and masculinity. One man who told his co-workers he was unable to have a child got— instead of sympathy—guffaws, *Playboy* magazines on his desk, and offers to teach him the "how-to's." Fear of such responses may even push a man to make his wife tell others it's her fault, maybe even to the point of deluding himself.[4]

To guard ourselves from such pressures, from unsolicited advice and nosy, painful questions, we can begin to cut ourselves off from those around us. Some couples radically change their life-styles to keep from being constantly reminded of how fertile everyone else seems to be. Some may leave jobs that involve contact with children, and some may move to a neighborhood not strewn with tricycles and soccer balls. Others may even quit attending church where the emphasis on family just reinforces their feelings of being "disfavored." And sadly, some couples may actually sever relations with family and friends to help ease the pain. In its worst form, that severing can also happen within marriage.

And even if you don't physically isolate yourselves, you can feel emotionally isolated. How else can you feel when you don't know which emotion will pop up next? Holidays depress you. You feel anger at the sight of the fifth baby this week paraded through your office. You feel sad in the middle of a group at a party. You're suddenly embarrassed as you realize you are telling a total stranger about your sperm antibody test. You find yourself fighting back tears in the grocery store line when your gaze falls on a magazine cover of a movie star and her new baby. Almost imperceptibly you may feel a sort of slow panic, thinking that no matter what you do it will be too late.

And to make matters worse, you begin to have a sort of philosophical crisis as you face the possibility of infertility, entertaining questions such as: "What's life about?" "What am I living for?" "What will I leave behind when I'm gone?" As your fertility crisis unfolds, it's disconcerting to find yourself doing, saying, thinking, dreaming—all in ways that seem beyond your control. Church shouldn't depress you. But it does. Family gatherings shouldn't make you sad. But they do. Toy trucks and baby seats and Sesame Street shouldn't make you cry, for goodness sake. But they do—at the weirdest times. And you begin to wonder if you're losing your mind.

But you're not. Everything you are feeling, someone else has felt—and someone else has worked through. There are stages all couples experiencing the uncertainty of an infertility work-up will go through—even if they *do* finally have a baby. And yet, society really has no way of helping us acknowledge that progression and come to terms with it.

The emotional stages of infertility have been likened to Elisabeth Kübler-Ross' stages of dying. First, the denial, then the rage, then bargaining, guilt, and depression. Then—if that long-sought-after baby is not born—grief and acceptance. Why would the stages of death be so relevant to the infertility crisis? Madeline Grupa, a Washington D.C. psychiatric nurse who works with infertile couples explains: ". . . [A] part of you dies when you cannot give birth to your own child. It is clearly a loss—a loss of a function of your body, or your genetic heritage, or a pregnancy, the loss of all the fantasies that go along with having a biological child."[5]

But infertility is still very much its own unique emotional experience. There's one big difference between it and a loved one's death. When a person loses someone through death, family and friends automatically rally around, comforting, supporting, bringing food and companionship, allowing that person the very natural opportunity to talk through the sense of loss and grief. But with the infertility crisis, no one—no one— may know what you're going through beyond your spouse and your doctor. And worse, except for the possible experience of miscarriage or stillbirth, there is no single moment to grieve, no specific time for your feelings to naturally surface. And the uncertainty can play havoc with your emotional state.

The book title of Barbara Berg's account of her own infertility expresses the situation more poignantly. It's entitled *Nothing to Cry About*. That phrase is one that any person going through the experience understands instantly. Its starkness and simplicity speak volumes about the frustrating, double-sided nature of the crisis. In one sense, the title is untrue. There is much to cry about. But in another, it is painfully true. How can you mourn the loss of someone who has never been born, and maybe never conceived? Since there is nothing tangible to represent the loss, the pain is hard to resolve, the loss hard to understand. As a Houston psychologist, Patricia Mahlstedt, put it: "There is much to cry about, and there is nothing to cry about. Everything is lost, and nothing is lost."[6]

Often couples battling infertility have likened their feelings to those of parents with a loved one missing in action—grief fenced in by hope. And the feeling seems to invade the rest of life. Such were one writer's feelings:

> At first my depression focused on never having children and missing the experience of pregnancy and childbirth. But as time

passed, it was as if the blockage in my tubes spread, clogging all the pathways of my body until I was inert. I was paralyzed by a low-grade joylessness. Part of the problem was the obsessive uncertainty of the loss. It was like having a son missing in action. Finally, like so many others, I longed not so much for pregnancy, but for resolution. Even if it meant giving up.[7]

The blow is hard for those who find out abruptly that they will never bear their own child. But infertility's worst impact is that numbing, ongoing, "anticipatory" sort of grief that comes when the treatment process is prolonged and unsuccessful. "Normal" infertile couples—those that seemingly have no medical reason for their infertility—and couples who have continual surgery or continual miscarriages know this sort of unspoken grief most of all. When the realization hits the couple battling infertility that their lives together are not turning out the way they planned, then the psychological effects begin to show up. As Mahlstedt sees it:

> They focus their attention on what they have failed to accomplish and soon start neglecting other goals and needs in their lives. . . . There is no balance in their lives. There is, instead, hope one week, grief the next. This cycle creates a very confusing roller coaster with depression, anger, and guilt as part of its down side.[8]

Much too often, couples float dizzily through the experience wishing for support and comfort from those around them. But with the infertility crisis, as opposed to other more visible crises in life, a couple will have to tell others about their situation and how they feel if they are to benefit from any possible support or comfort. And that takes an awareness of what is happening to them psychologically, and, very possibly, a tremendous leap over such emotional hurdles as embarrassment and anger and fear. Sadly, but understandably, some couples never make the leap. In citing the quiet jeopardy of the infertility crisis, Barbara Menning points out this danger: "Since there may be repeated crisis states during infertility investigation and treatment, there is the very real risk of maladaptive behavioral changes, just as there is the real chance for positive growth and increased insight."[9]

Tragically, most couples may not have any way to know that their feelings are very normal and very common. They may wonder if they are going to end up not only childless, but alienated from friends and family, in divorce court, or in some sort of suspended sexual conflict for the rest of their marriage.[10] But the good news is that these feelings *are* felt by others, and like others, the painful tense feelings *can* mend—with a little openness, a little knowledge, and a little time.

To help with the awareness any couple needs to leap those hurdles toward positive growth and openness, we should explore the predictable stages any of us going through an infertility crisis may experience.

THE EMOTIONAL STAGES OF INFERTILITY

What are these predictable stages? And how do they fit into our experience? The order and depth of these feelings may vary, and so will the speed with which they are resolved, but you as a couple and as individuals will probably feel them all, at one time or another.

DENIAL

Most often, the couple who has been faced with possible infertility will begin by denying the possibility that a problem exists. The whole idea seems crazy. Like everyone else, you probably spent years doing your best to keep pregnancy from happening. Then you may have worked your lives around the idea of children by taking less demanding jobs or living in certain places just to accommodate that impending family. And now. . . . Nothing you've been taught has prepared you for even the possibility of infertility. RESOLVE founder Barbara Menning was quite surprised how many people she counseled said they could have accepted infertility more readily if only they had known how common it is.

So at first we're surprised, and we experience denial of even the thought of not being fertile. And though initial denial is healthy, intended to be a short-term coping mechanism to help ease a person into the realization of a crisis, it's never meant to be a solution to the crisis.[11] Often a person just cannot handle the "label" of infertility—even its possibility in his or her life—perhaps due to its seeming threat to sexuality. Out of fear, such a person may drop out or never start a medical work-up, and will become "stuck" in his/her denial. This sort of prolonged denial can not only be dangerous, but obviously self-defeating. "Prolonged denial may take such forms as a declaration that such matters are 'in God's hands' or up to Mother Nature. The longer a problem is denied, without resolution, the less realistic the denial becomes and the more emotional effort the denial demands," states Judith Stigger in her book, *Coping with Infertility*.[12]

And such emotional output may take its toll in unexpected ways. Stigger tells the story of Jo Ann who, after several years of trying to have a baby, suddenly denied any problem. Declaring that such matters were up to God, she refused to seek medical help. Meanwhile, though, babies became an obsession with her. She even kept a list of fifty carefully chosen baby names in her purse. Yet she suppressed all anger and doubt, becoming more and more emotionally exhausted and more and more detached from reality.

Then after six years, Jo Ann had a baby. And everything was fine . . . right? Wrong. "By then," Stigger explains, "containing those unresolved feelings had destroyed her ability to respond to new events in her life. She could not cope with the demands of parenting. Seven months later she abandoned her husband and her baby and never returned."[13]

Such a dramatic story sounds so drastic, so unbelievable. But we really don't know the extent of the power our emotions have over us. The only healthy denial is initial denial. And that's the kind that almost all couples will go through before they can move on, before they *must* move on. Different people, though, will experience initial denial in different ways.

One form of denial is to recognize the possibility of a problem but not to accept the responsibility of it, giving it to spouse or doctor or God or fate. "It's my husband's fault," or "God is just testing us," or "The doctor will find out what's wrong," or "It's just not our time yet."

In yet another form of denial, the "can-do" spirit takes over. The quest will be for a "cure." If there's a problem, well, surely it can be fixed: "Some expert somewhere has the answer." "Maybe if I try those herbs my aunt gave me." "If I do exactly what the doctor says. . . ." Sometimes this denial manifests itself in a form of bargaining, as one woman explains it:

> If I were a very good girl, did exactly what I was told, endured pain and embarrassment without complaint, then I would be rewarded. Somehow I believed that the act of dutifully taking my temperature every day for 365 days would actually trigger fertilization.[14]

The sort of personality you have will greatly influence how you respond at this stage—and for that matter, to the crisis as a whole. If you are the type that tends to "go with the flow," you'll do the same with infertility. If you are a self-motivator, you'll be one through this crisis. One friend, a very positive go-getter, when asked by her husband what she would do if they didn't have a baby, listed her plan of attack as: *(1) natural pregnancy, (2) A.I.H. (Artificial Insemination by Husband), (3) A.I.D. (Artificial Insemination by Donor), (4) adoption, (5) in vitro fertilization,* and, *if all else fails—(6) kidnapping at the grocery store.*

Most responses have their built-in advantages. A positive, "can-do" attitude comes in very handy in keeping the medical work-up "blues" at bay, for instance. The "go-with-the-flow" type may find the stress easier to take, because he or she naturally fends off most anxiety and tension. But many responses have built-in dangers, too. The plodding, systematic type will carry on, but may find feelings of depression and anxiety overwhelming. The go-getters, for all their energy, may find the going tougher when the medical work-up goes on and on. In such a situation, these high-achievers who feel they can overcome any obstacle if they just put their minds and energy to it may be stunned by the awful helplessness that ultimately hits them. Psychiatrist Miriam Mazor has found:

> The go-getters continue to be go-getters and have a hard time knowing when to quit. [And] those people who generally feel like victims of fate in other areas of their life will probably not approach infertility aggressively enough, will not push hard enough and will keep bungling along with the same doctor.[15]

If the "cure" can't be found by physical means, then maybe you might begin thinking the problem is emotional or mental. You might begin believing that it is "all in your head." Family, friends, even doctors may hint at such. "Try to relax," they may say. "Maybe you're trying to hard." When a doctor suggested this sort of thing to one woman, she blew up: "I told him that if he thought I was uptight, he should meet my mother! My grandmother was even worse, and she had eight children. I come from a long line of uptight fertile women!"[16]

If a couple finds out about their "absolute" infertility abruptly, as with a sterile sperm test or sudden hysterectomy, the denial will set in quickly but usually end quickly, allowing the couple to grieve in a healthy way. But most infertility is revealed methodically, through a long list of tests and treatments that may or may not be clear. And then denial may tag along, becoming unhealthy if given too much time.

Through these first few denial responses, a serious by-product may be isolation—not just from others such as family or friends, but even from each other. The wife may be frustrated with the husband's inability to show enthusiasm for the medical work-up. He may not be listening anymore when she talks about it, especially if she is constantly talking about it in hopes of getting some response from him. He may, likewise, be anxious over sperm tests and sex on demand. Isolation within the marriage is not unusual, as the medical work-up becomes a daily, stress-filled part of their lives. But when allowing each other "space" to cope becomes a total, lingering lack of communication, it is obviously a very unhealthy sign.

Denial *will* come and go, though, even after you've effectively trudged on into other stages. I found this to be true only a few days ago, as I waited for another ultrasound. The technician was explaining to a nurse in the room that I was an infertile patient, and this was an ultrasound for my treatment. I winced. I had just been labeled as "infertile," and I didn't like it. I didn't like the sound of it, the bland, unattractive, barren sound of the word. And I especially didn't like it being attached to me. Part of my feeling was the curse of being a "normal" infertile couple for so long. I still wanted to believe this was all a big mistake. But for that instant, I *denied* it all—until I realized how crazy and off-base the feeling was, and let it go.

But even though the feelings of denial may surface from time to time, and even though the effects of the denial—the isolation, the questions, the "cure" attempts, even the dreams and fantasies about pregnancy—may linger, denial *will* melt into other stages.

ANGER

Soon, the "No, not me," becomes the "Why me?" Anger very naturally sets in. The anger may be rational—focused on real things like tests or treatments. Or it may be irrational—targeting doctors, spouses, God, abortion rights advocates, or anyone who seems to have control over pregnancy.

An easy target is the *doctor*. One woman describes her first visit to her specialist in terms that may sound all too familiar. "Dr. C." greeted her impersonally from behind a massive desk strewn with folders. Everything in the office seemed offensive: the tiny birth-control pill encased in a Plexiglas paperweight

("I'd taken them for five years," she realized. "Had they been the culprit?"); the framed needlepoint of Dr. C. delivering a baby, a handmade gift from a satisfied customer ("Would I too come to worship this cool professional as my savior?"); the photograph of Dr. C's gorgeous wife and teenage daughters smiling broadly and squinting from the glare atop the deck of a sailboat ("Would we have a carefree family outing? Would a sunny day ever seem so bright?") Nothing seemed right, and as she explained it: ". . . I wasn't at all certain I'd come to the right place, but as I left the office, I felt sure of one thing: I'd found someone to blame. For the better part of a year, Dr. C. would be my most intimate enemy."[17]

Another easy target is the *spouse*. One husband felt it deeply: "In some of our knock-down, drag-out fights, she has yelled, 'You can't even make a child.' That cuts me down to nothing."[15] Also, a wife may fault her husband for not being willing to carry more of her emotional burden: "He says he understands my feelings and sympathizes, but doesn't care to hear any more about the subject."[19]

It's a good bet, though, that however both of you are coping, you're not coping at the same speed or the same place. You can easily push one another away emotionally just because the two of you are reacting differently to the same crisis. You may attempt to respond in a loving way about the crisis and yet be totally misunderstood by your spouse. Two of my friends found this to be painfully true. Trying to let his wife know he valued her above everything, one night he said to her, "So what if we don't ever have children? It doesn't matter." *She* replied by throwing a cold drink in his face. Because she was emotionally on a very different level than her husband, she interpreted his remark as an insensitive wish to quit or to downplay the situation's importance. You can imagine what he thought.

But such situations are not unusual. Feelings are raw, nerves are on edge, communication is at a record low. You, the wife, may be in much more despair over testing than your husband, while you, the husband, may feel hurt by your wife's openness with others about intimate details. Or vice-versa. Because both of you are doing your own emotional juggling, neither of you may have what it takes to help one another, and that is when you turn to others for help.

. . . which brings us to *friends and family.* You can easily find yourself angry with those around you because you feel they can't seem to comfort you or relate to your problem. They might not be able to understand your depression or helplessness and only offer perfunctory pep-talks such as "Wait till next month," or "It'll happen. Give it time." Their lack of sympathy and their insensitive remarks ("Hey, need a lesson or two? (wink, wink)," "Haven't you got a bun in the oven yet?") can make you feel unloved, unaccepted, misunderstood, even ashamed. No relationship can stand up under that sort of strain.

And many of those remarks seem to come out of nowhere, when you least expect it. When the husband of one of my friends heard we had bought a water bed, he made several crass comments—in a group—about the bed helping our "cause." He was trying to be funny. No one laughed. And I wanted to punch his lights out. Instead, I smiled weakly and my husband shrugged it off.

Strangely enough, people who make such remarks probably don't even know they've hurt you, and if you haven't confided in them, they may not even know you're hurting. Yet it's a vicious circle, because even if you do confide in them they may not be able to give you what you need. And you end up feeling bewildered, mad, and even humiliated by how you act around them—and paranoid about what will happen next.

One friend tells of holding her baby niece as she had so many times before, talking the usual amount of baby-talk to the infant, when suddenly she realized she had said, "Mama loves you . . . yes she does," within earshot of her sister-in-law, the baby's mother. She almost choked. Without a word, she handed the baby to her sister-in-law and walked out of the room, dumbfounded and embarrassed by the slip of her tongue.

Such painful situations can be the cause of many couples' pulling away from others. It's easier to retreat than to show your anger outwardly. Isolating yourself sometimes comes from a need for self-preservation, a need to protect privacy, dignity, or self-image. Opening up to others is a big risk. You may be disappointed at their lack of understanding. You'll expect too much, maybe, from these important people in your life, your anger will well up—and you'll keep your distance. But interestingly enough, you may be surprised by understanding and comfort from unexpected sources. One person here or there may know exactly why you're reticent to answer that nosy question, or another may just notice your sad mood and want to talk. Being open to these moments may be just what you need.

Anger can also be aimed at *yourself*. This can take many forms, one being the effect it has on your *self-image*. If you're an otherwise calm, rational person, and yet you find yourself out of control, you'll wonder what hit you. My first talk with my new boss began normallly enough, calmly enough. But when he asked me about my plans for the future, all I could think about was the specialist I was going to see and the medical work-up I was going through—and I couldn't hold back the tears. I had never broken down in front of my doctor, rarely cried with my friends or even my family, and, yet, there I was bawling my eyes out in front of the vice-president of my division. I don't think I have ever been so mad at myself, mad at my lack of control, and mad at the preoccupation my fertility quest had assumed over my life. It was seeping into every area of my life, and I didn't much like the person it was turning me into.

Self-image plays a drastic part in the emotional crisis of possible infertility. If you have a healthy self-image, you will weather this emotional crisis better, quicker, easier. Just like a person in good physical condition bounces back from illness better, so will a person in this situation who feels valued for other things. In your marriage, if you feel of value despite the infertility, if you are wanted and loved for more than your procreation talents, then you'll realize you're worthy of the love of your spouse no matter what your physical flaws. If your family and friends affirm you for yourself, you'll make the passage quicker, whether you become pregnant or not.

If your self-esteem is already low, though, anger turned inward may drop it to the pits. You may begin believing you are not worthy of having a child. You may seriously wonder if your spouse would be better off without you. Bargaining or a sort of atonement may follow in which you might try to do anything to make up for the "cause," including volunteering for experimental procedures, or jumping into donor artificial insemination or in vitro fertilization or adoption—anything to get a child and make everything all right.

People who have difficulty expressing anger can't help but feel confused, not knowing how to respond. You can't forget those childhood lessons that taught us that "good" people don't get angry, jealous, or resentful, and so guilt sets in further.[16] Those with an internal sense of justice will feel betrayed and angry at the humiliation they feel through no fault of their own. Couples going through "secondary infertility" (in which they are unable to have a second child) often feel angry at themselves, seeing themselves as being selfish or self-indulgent for wanting another child when they already have one.

If denied, the anger can be displaced, taking such forms as guilt or depression, tension headaches or testiness. You might try the "Count your blessings" approach, or the "Get a hold of yourself—you haven't got a good reason for self-pity" angle. Or even the "Buck up, life's not so bad" routine.

But not *accepting* your *right* to your anger will only boomerang, even to the extent of changing your personality. Such was the case with one of Dr. Mahlstedt's patients:

> My husband told me he hated what the past few years had done to me. He said he watched me turn into an angry, bitter,

hateful person. It was a long time before I realized how angry I was. I was *consumed* with anger before I understood what was eating me up inside. Then my problem was finding what to do with my anger—how at least to channel it, if not resolve it.[21]

GUILT

If the in-grown anger takes the form of guilt, you may begin asking yourself questions such as: Did we wait too long: Did I bring this on myself? Are we doing something wrong now? Is this some sort of punishment? "WHAT DID I DO TO DESERVE THIS?" we want to yell. We grope for a reason. If an understandable reason can just be found, we think, we'd feel less frustrated, less angry, less depressed.

The past can easily become a factor, a debilitating one in the guilt scheme. Premarital sex, extramarital sex, abortions, venereal disease, anything considered bad in one's past is dredged up and reexamined, especially if there is good reason to believe it may have had an effect on fertility.[22]

The *past* can play another part, too. Infertility can be such a blow to self-esteem that even childhood traumas you've thought you'd outgrown can surface. Don't be surprised if you're suddenly reminded of other failures, those that helped shape your self-esteem during your delicate adolescent days— anything from being too fat, to being too tall, to being rejected by a club or a group or a team or a special person, to being poor, to being a late bloomer, to having a physical handicap, to being of the "wrong" race or social class. There's a trauma for every adolescent that ever lived. And even though they may sound minor now, they were major then—and that's the hurt and the image you may carry into adulthood. Every one of them is connected in some way to self-image, self-esteem, and sexuality—the very issues infertility touches most personally. There really is no preventing those old issues from coming back to haunt you in this adult crisis. And in some cases, those old issues left painfully unresolved may have to be coped with first before you can cope with your present problem. Just being aware of *why* they've surfaced may help.

DEPRESSION

Anger turned inward usually produces some sort of depression. This has to be the most common reaction to the infertility. Every reminder of your childless state—a baby shower invitation, a neighbor's kid scooting down the sidewalk, the pregnant mannequin in the front window of the maternity shop at the mall—can instantly depress you. And the sense of helplessness with each new test of the medical work-up can be devastating. Highs and lows are the words to describe the emotional seesaw the medical situation puts you on—highs when some therapy seems to be working and you are encouraged, and then lows when the next cycle comes and you're not pregnant. Slowly, depression sets in as a way of life. For some, the longing is overwhelming. No day goes by without thinking about it, no activity unmarred, no prayer unburdened by that gnawing sense of empty longing.

For some, depressive episodes are periodic and brief—starting each day plotting your temperature chart is enough to make anyone depressed. Others learn to live with it, like carrying around so much extra emotional baggage. And still others find depression the last straw, allowing it to immobilize them from everyday life. As one woman watched her life slowly change, she realized: "Life contains little joy. I worried that I did not laugh anymore."[23]

This brings up a serious side effect of coping with a seemingly never-ending crisis. So much of your emotional energy is being used in the attempt to keep some sort of emotional equilibrium that there is no energy left for anything else. Because low-grade depression leaves you feeling drained and lifeless, vulnerable to any other crisis that might come your way, you very easily may not have any strength left to cope with it. Being aware of this danger may help you divert such a situation by reaching out for help if and when other crises hit.

In her study of the psychological aspects of infertility, Dr. Patricia Mahlstedt explains that infertility creates many simultaneous and complex losses. The phenomenon of so many losses coupled with so little outlet for support or grief, leads to intense stress. "Like loss, stress depletes people of psychological energy ordinarily used to enjoy life and to solve problems of all magnitude. Less able to cope, people become depressed."[24]

Recent research into depression categorizes the losses in adulthood that are definite factors in depression. *Loss of relationship, loss of health, loss of status or prestige, loss of self-esteem, loss of self-confidence, loss of security, loss of fantasy or the hope of fulfilling an important fantasy, or loss of something or someone of great symbolic value*—any *one* of these can cause depression in an adult.[25] And as Mahlstedt ironically points out, the experience of infertility involves ALL of them. So, our possible reactions to each of these are worthy of note:

Loss of relationship takes its form in the isolation you feel from your spouse, your family and friends, the ever-fertile world. It's a kind of "unspoken fear." Will my spouse leave me if we can't have our own natural children? Is my depression driving everyone away? Will my friends with kids find less and less time for us?

With all the emotional strain and drain, the timed sex, the demands made, and the needs unmet, even the closest couple will begin to feel worlds apart. Too easily, any couple can begin to resent each other and become depressed, not only because they are having trouble conceiving but also because they feel the loss of closeness and understanding.

The very normal drifting away of your friends with kids cuts deeply. Unconsciously they may leave you out as they begin to base most of their activities around their children, doing things that they may think you wouldn't be interested in. That reality came home to me one rare snowy Texas Sunday as two friends of mine were talking about how much fun they had had on Saturday. They'd had a terrific time pulling the kids—

and themselves—on a sled behind their cars up and down their street. I stood there wondering why they hadn't called us over to get in on the fun. And then I knew why. It was kid's fun . . . or at least fun that adults have because they happen to have kids. It never occurred to them we might have loved it too. I don't think I ever felt more alone, more unconsciously rejected than at that moment. And I wondered if our infertility would be the death of our friendships.

As for "unspoken" fears, any person of devout faith will find the most unspeakable of all may be a confused, untouchable anxiety—a fear of facing feelings about God and his place in this crisis. Such a possible rift in this relationship touches the very essence of a person of faith's being, calling into question his or her whole spiritual frame of reference. (Section 5 discusses this tension in detail.)

Loss of health encompasses how we feel about our bodies. With every trip to the doctor and the hospital, you might begin to slowly view your body as damaged or defective, and possibly unattractive. Something is obviously wrong, you think, and so your image of your body changes. Uncomfortable and sometimes unsuccessful treatment, undignified positions, and even experimental medications can make anyone susceptible to a poor "body image."[26] Just the idea that your body will not do what you had always thought it could do, is a shock. As one woman shared, "My expectations of myself are changing. I once had the expectation that my body would do almost anything that I wanted it to do, not necessarily instantly, but certainly with perseverance and training. . . ."[27] Finding out that your body may have unforeseen limitations can be a blow. There is a true loss of physical possibilities, and you cannot escape the strange feeling of seeing yourself in a different way.

The medical work-up experience alone can do funny things to your head. I realized after several years that I was actually thinking of myself as somehow "sick". I knew I was healthy. Test after test after test had hold me how normal I was. But for a normal, healthy person, I sure was going to the doctor a lot. And very few normal, healthy people I knew had blood drawn every other month or so. Consciously I knew myself to be in good health, but subconsciously I wasn't quite sure.

For those who pride themselves in being in good physical shape, a "kink" in one's "body image" may be hard to take. And the reaction may be to overcompensate. I have always been an athletically inclined yet somewhat lazy person. But in the last few years, I have made a inspired effort to be in good shape—to the extent of becoming a slow but diligent runner, an avid racquetball player, and even a decent swimmer. I feel better physically than I have ever felt in my life. I'm in better shape than I have ever been in my life.

Yet lately I've begun wondering if my recent preoccupation with fitness may be a reaction to my experience with needles and pills and examination rooms. At first I used exercise to relieve the stress I was feeling, and it still does that. But now I realize that over these last few years, the same years I've been on the infertility grind, I have been much more aware of my body and how it feels and looks than I ever had been before.

As obsessions go, I suppose it is one of the healthier ones, but overdoing anything can still be detrimental. So my awareness of this normal reaction helps me keep a possible obsession in check.

In a very real way, though, there may be an actual loss of health. "The cumulative effect of the entire process of diagnosis and treatment can lead to physical illness," Mahlstedt believes.[28] The stress of the depression and other strong emotions can be the cause of all sorts of physical problems: poor sleeping and eating habits, upset stomach, headaches, ulcers, not to mention such self-defeating problems as bouts of impotence and disrupted menstrual cycles. The side effects of some medications alone can make you feel awful.

Some people may actually bring on a loss of health through forms of self-destructiveness, especially if poor self-esteem is a factor. In her counseling, Barbara Menning has dealt with several cases of drug abuse, alcoholism, anorexia, and obesity that were obvious examples of the "maladaptive behaviorial changes" she warns about. And in each case, the infertility work had to be postponed until the patient's health was restored and the behavior readjusted—which is never an easy or quick task.

Also, there's no ignoring the fact that some of the infertility testing and therapies require surgical procedures, which, of course, include the hazard of going under anaesthesia. I'll never forget my first realization of this danger. Lying on a table waiting to undergo a laparascopy, I was nervously contemplating the ceiling tiles when I was rudely reminded of my mortality. A nurse leaned over, pushed pen and paper under my nose, and matter-of-factly instructed me to read and sign a form about the possibility of my never waking up again. I remember nearly hopping off that table and heading for the door. And I also remember wondering, angrily, why this very basic part of surgery had not been pointed out to me before that critical, emotional point.

The effect your body image has on the sexual side of your marriage cannot be ignored, either. Infertility will inevitably take a toll on sex. Making babies replaces making love. The demand to perform can only deaden your image of yourself and your image of how the one you love sees you. And the result may be that you begin worrying that sex will never be special again, that infertility has ruined this part of your relationship. And being told otherwise is little comfort.

Loss of status or prestige is a direct result of the obvious worth our society places on parenthood. Is there any doubt of this fact? A quick thought back to the last time someone asked you how many kids you had will remove that doubt. And this status situation seems harder for the woman since she has been groomed subliminally since birth for the role of "mother." We are programmed to procreate, it seems. But we as infertile couples aren't following the program. And worse, society expects us to or demands to know why we aren't!

In many ways, even our own sexual identities may become

fogged. Our concepts of masculinity and femininity, whether we like it or not, are quite entangled with fertility and virility. Add our present-day emphasis on family life and effective parenting, and it's easy to see why society makes its children forms of status. And so once again, we feel . . . different, like we don't belong, like we've lost the respect and acceptance, somehow, of our "group." Picture your high school reunion, that bastion of last chance status-seeking. After my first reunion, I left convinced that if I had told every old classmate of mine that I had written the #1 bestseller in the country, won a Pulitzer prize for it, and had just sold the rights for the movie, most of them would have responded with, "That's nice. Have any children?" and proceed to show me baby pictures.

To be so out of "sync" with our peers hurts. Nothing we accomplish will seem good enough as long as we place a high value on what others think. And it's very hard not to.

Loss of self-esteem involves the idea mentioned earlier. Our pride—how we in effect view ourselves—can be damaged as we find we may not become what we've envisioned ourselves as becoming, doing what we've always thought we had within our powers to do, being what we believe others want us to be. The inevitable questions about our "maleness" or "femaleness," concepts integral to anyone's self-image, may pop up. "What kind of woman/man am I if I can't even produce a child?" we may wonder as we lie awake at night.

Loss of self-confidence is due to loss of control. Despite the huge price you pay in terms of money, time, persistence, commitment, and sacrifice, you can't do what everyone else seems to do with the smallest amount of effort. "I can't have a baby? Anybody—everybody—can have a baby!" Also, a couple can easily become overwhelmed with the choices they face: "When do I stop taking medication? Having surgery? Or keeping temperature charts?" "Am I a quitter if I do?" "Should I change doctors?" "Should we adopt?" "Should we remain childless?" "Should we consider these new procedures?" All those serious choices, brought on by a situation you never asked for, may actually shut down your decision-making capacity for a time. Confidence in yourself and your ability to cope may take a nose-dive straight into depression.

Loss of security entails the damage the infertility crisis can have on jobs, such as time missed or promotions turned down because you hesitate moving in the middle of a treatment, or on marriage, when you worry how your relationship is being affected. Plus, the financial burden of infertility can take its toll, easily eating up any extra money you might have, even if you are insured.

And on a deeper level, there's also loss of security over the fairness of life. If this can happen, you think, then anything could happen. And that is one scary thought, especially if we've always felt life is supposed to ultimately work out for the better.

Loss of fantasy means loss of a dream. All of us have had those ideas of our future that included all the trappings of parenthood—being pregnant, giving birth, baby's first step, first day of school, wedding day, graduation, grandchildren—the list is endless. Having a child is tantamount to growing up and becoming a true adult for many, many people. And whether we would ever have listed parenting as the dream of our future, we probably would admit we had always seen it as being a part of that future. The possibility of losing that vision can hurt deeply. We may wonder what *will* fill the future. Will it be lonely? Will it be empty? Will it be . . . happy?

Loss of something or someone of great symbolic value. I don't think it will come as a surprise to anyone going through the experience of infertility that the "dream child" you've consciously or unconsciously envisioned has been a sort of symbol of the future. Any such symbol has much psychological value to a human being. This loss may be felt most dramatically in your marriage, where one of the important aspects of shared parenting is surely the feeling that the child is *yours*, symbolic of your love and "oneness." With the possibility you may not have your own "flesh and blood" child goes a loss of personal continuity—the feeling that a part of both of your lives would live on in your child. The potential loss of such a deeply-felt symbol of the future demands a restructuring, maybe a reconstructing of a whole new value structure.[29]

Denial, anger, guilt, depression—it's an emotional roller coaster ride for sure. Yet, roller coaster rides come to an end. They must come to an end. And when this one does, it's time for grief—which may be the most elusive emotion of the lot.

GRIEF

As a stage in the infertility experience, grief is hard to pigeonhole. There are couples who give up, dropping out of the medical work-up early, who may never truly face their loss in a healthy way. But in other infertile couples' experience, two things will eventually take place. Either a pregnancy happens, and the debris of the emotional aspects of infertility slowly disappears, or the final treatments come about and they are forced to face the situation squarely.

You'd think that grief would begin at that point. But that's not always the case. Grief begins only with a moment of clearly perceived loss. In "absolute infertility," when there is no hope, the moment of loss is very clear. But in most cases of infertility, there really isn't a clear ending. Because there could always be one more test, one more specialist to try, the moment of grieving is elusive.

This inability to grieve is the single most common problem Barbara Menning has encountered in all her years of counseling infertile couples. When infertility includes stillbirth or miscarriage, the couple is forced to focus on a specific loss, and will experience more normal grieving—for a time, at least. But for the couple caught up in the usual fertility quest, a normal sort of grieving may not materialize because the loss is an invisible one. It's a loss of potential, not of an actual object. The quest carries with it a sort of "grief-on-hold," an on-going, numbing sort of grief you keep pushing back, pushing back. And because of this innate sort of defensive reflex, a healthy grief process may be possible only when the couple, yearning for resolution, as mentioned before, choose to experience it by ending the testing themselves.

However you arrive at the grief stage, though, you must allow yourself to feel it. The fear of letting go, of being out of control has to be thrown aside. Your grief, at some point, must be taken off hold and allowed to wash over you. Then, just like other experiences you've had with grief, this grief *will* come to an end.

A healthy grief process will pave the way to *resolution,* a form of acceptance that is the ultimate goal of any such crisis. That's not to say you won't ever again feel these emotions. You will. According to the experiences of the many couples she's worked with, Barbara Menning explains you will feel them only occasionally, but they won't ever again be as controlling or overwhelming. And you'll handle them with a quiet strength, because they'll be brief, and you'll be able to cope with them philosophically.

How does it feel when your grief is resolved? According to some people who've been through it, the feeling could be somewhat like this:

> There is a return of energy, perhaps even a surge of zest and well-being; a sense of perspective emerges; optimism and faith return and also a sense of humor—and some past absurdities may even become grist for storytelling; self-image is again perceived correctly . . . self-esteem returns (good things can happen to me; I deserve to do well); sexuality can be forever disconnected from thoughts of childbearing and enjoyed in its own right, for its own sake. Plans for the future can be made again with confidence.[30]

Now you know what to expect. You may have already identified yourself in this section's pages. But knowing where you are may not be enough to change how you feel. That may be impossible right now. You *must* feel the way you do. It's only natural. What these pages should do is work on your awareness of where you are, with an eye to what you will probably feel next. And then—when you are ready, they should help lead you through the stages in a healthy, positive way. You can't push yourself through these stages any more than you can control those crazy emotions you're feeling. You can, though, realize if you are being stuck on one of them in an unhealthy way.

But giving a name to all the emotions you're feeling, realizing you're stuck, even being told what's probably coming next, doesn't help you do much about it. And that's probably what you want to know most of all—how to cope, how to break out of the emotional stronghold. In other words, what to *do* . . . .

"Hey you two!" one of our friends calls to us as we get out of our car. "Long time no see! Want some watermelon? Homemade ice cream? Got some chocolate chip over here!"

"Best picnic I've been to in a long time," one guy is saying as he stuffs his mouth with homemade pie.

"You mean best free food, Denny. We all know you," another friend says, then turns to us. "Hey, everybody, look who's here!"

"Wellllll, you two haven't been to one of these get-togethers in a long time. Get some ice cream! Have a seat!" Denny suggests magnanimously.

"Make it two scoops," my husband is saying to the older woman dishing out the strawberry ice cream.

"No, Shawn," Denny's wife is telling their six-year-old, "you cannot go over to the tennis courts. You'll bug the players. Je-re-my!? Here, Denny hold the baby for a minute. Where is that Jeremy?" She gets up and walks through a circle of young women, most of them either feeding babies or corralling toddlers. "Has anyone seen Jeremy? Oooh, that boy."

One of the women is feeding her baby some ice cream: "C'mon, darling, open wide. This is goooood." The baby lets out a howl.

"Oooh. Great pair of lungs," someone quips. And all the women laugh while the baby's mother tries to calm him.

One of the young mothers comes over and sits down beside me, baby in her arms. "Missed you at Donna's shower a few weeks ago. When are you two gonna get in on all this fun?" she smiles, glancing back at the ring of babies.

"Someday, probably," I smile back. "Any peach ice cream left?" I ask, and move toward the ice cream freezers all lined up on the picnic table. The lady scooping up the peach ice cream recognizes me as one of her daughter's classmates. "Lynda Rutledge, where have you been *hiding? It's so good to see you. Have I talked to you since Sherry's had her little girl? That was one BIG baby. She had to have a C-section. She's doing fine, though. It's her third, you know. And she thought she'd never have any. She'll be so glad to hear I've seen you. How are you? And your handsome husband? How many children do you have now?"*

"Oh none yet, Mrs. Jackson, but we . . . uh. None yet." I smile and nod at her as I turn to go. "Please tell Sherry hello for me. And congratulations."

"Thank you, dear. And I will certainly do that!"

"LYNDA! How are you?" I hear a familiar voice call from behind me.

"Well, hello! I haven't seen you in a long time. You and Scott still seeing each other?"

"It has been a long time!" she chuckles. "We're married, and I'm expecting! Say, when are you two gonna have a baby?"

"Oh, I dunno, how about next Tuesday?" I answer. We both laugh; she waves goodbye, and I move back to the picnic table where my husband and several others are sitting. My husband gets up, empty bowl in hand. "Be right back," he grins, as I sit down.

"Hey, girl," Denny says to me as he bounces his toddler on his knee, "you two are really missing out, not having kids. Are you ever going to get your act together?"

"Go ahead, Denny, ask me a personal question," I answer, as I stick a spoonful of ice cream in my mouth.

"Well, if you need any pointers . . . let me know (leer leer)."

I ignore him and eat another spoonful.

"Yeah, I tell ya," he continues, leaning closer, "you just gotta tell your ol' man to quit shooting you blanks."

The ice cream almost sticks in my throat, and I swallow hard, catching my breath. "That's not funny, Denny," I say, glaring across the table at him.

"Well, don't get all excited. Good grief. Can't you take a joke?"

"I mean it, Denny."

"Oh, c'mon!"

My husband walks up. I start to take another bite of my ice cream, then set the spoon down, feeling the heat rising up my neck. "I need to go home," I murmur to my husband as I grab my purse and head for the car. "Excuse me, everyone."

"WHAT is going ON?" my husband asks, trailing along behind me.

"Nothing. I just want to go home. Did you hear what Denny said? I felt like smacking him one!"

"Oh, it couldn't be that bad, honey."

"I'm just tired of it. We shouldn't have come." I get in the car and bang the car door shut behind me.

"We can't just hide, you know," he replies as he turns the ignition and pulls slowly away from the park. Neither of us say anything, riding the rest of the way home in silence.

As we pull into the driveway, he turns to me. "Are you going to tell me what happened or not?"

I look at him a moment, then gaze back out the window. "The other day, I met this woman. Nobody special, just someone I happened to meet. She asked me if I had any children—like everybody does. Not really interested. You know, just the thing to say. Well, I proceeded to unload on her. I told her my whole life story. I mean everything! Every detail! As if I had to justify not doing my part or something! She was a total stranger!"

My husband stifles a laugh.

"It's not funny," I mumble.

"I know. I was just picturing the lady's face."

"Yeah, well, she didn't hang around too long after that. Understandably."

"Why do you let it bother you so?" he asks me. "Whatever Denny said, you know he didn't mean anything."

"Nobody means anything. The normal remarks are hard enough to handle, but the crude ones . . ." I shake my head. "I shoulda smacked him one. I'd feel better."

My husband grins. "Lynda, just blow him off. He's harmless."

I turn my head abruptly back to him. "It's not like it's the first time, you know. Do you think he'd like you making crass sexual remarks to his wife?"

"Well, no . . . but that's just the way he is."

"So, I'm supposed to put up with stuff like that? I mean, you don't even see it," I go on, gesturing helplessly.

"Let's don't start this again."

"See?! Can't you see we keep ducking the situation?"

"No, we don't. We're okay," he replies.

I take a deep breath from somewhere in the pit of my stomach, and then slowly let it out. "It's affecting us," I reply quietly as I open my car door and get out.

"I think we're doing okay," he repeats, following me toward the house.

"It can't help but affect us," I mumble as I reach to open the front door.

"We're not that bad . . . We're OKAY," he says quietly yet firmly, as he places his hand tightly over mine on the doorknob.

I gaze up at him. "Honey, saying things are okay doesn't make it so. The last couple of years have been tense, and you know it."

"You're making too big a deal out of all this, and you know it," he answers, exasperated. We stand there, not moving, silent for a moment. Finally, he murmurs, "I . . . just don't want you to be upset so much."

"I don't want to be upset. I just . . . feel alone in this." I look back at him. "We need to talk. . . ."

He lowers his hand. "All right then. Let's talk. What do you think I'm doing wrong?"

"You're not listening. You're not seeing."

"Okay," he frowns. "You're probably right. Now," he goes on, "ask me what you're doing wrong."

"What."

"You're taking everything—and I mean everything—too personally."

I cross my arms, let out a long sigh, and then look at him sideways. "Maybe so."

It was his turn to sigh. Crossing his arms too, he leaned heavily on the door. "Look, things could be a lot worse, you know."

"Oh yeah, how?"

"You could be married to Denny."

We both burst out laughing, and then he pulls me close, hugging tight.

"Never," *I declare, pulling back a little.* "And anyway, I wouldn't want to have his kid."

"I think there's a compliment in there somewhere," *my husband mutters, pulling me close again.* "So. What do you want to do about our friends?"

"I don't know," *I shrug, resting my chin on his shoulder, suddenly very tired.* "But I do know I don't want to tell every little personal detail to everybody we know."

"Like the lady?"

"Like the lady."

Right then, as if on cue, the telephone rings. Opening the door, my husband glances toward the sound. "You know who that probably is. You want me to answer it?"

"No, I suppose I should," *I reply, moving toward the phone.*

"What are you going to say to him?"

"I don't know. I'll think of something—but no more crude jokes. No more." *And I pick up the phone.*

HOW DO I COPE?

The Social Crisis

"Do you think we're pregnant?" Over the years we've been married, I've posed that question several times to my husband. . .

. . . when I was twenty-two and forgot to take my birth control pill, I asked it apprehensively.

. . . when I was twenty-eight and ready to start a family, I asked it hopefully.

. . . when I was thirty-one and in the midst of our fertility testing, I asked it anxiously.

. . . and last month, as I turned 35, I leaned across a restaurant table and asked it jokingly. My husband cocked an eyebrow, the people at the next table stopped in mid-chew, and my husband and I both laughed. The question had become one of our all-time inside jokes. But my way of coping.

Coping? I suppose that's what I've been doing with that omnipresent question for most of my adult life. That question and all the other questions that go with it. Humor is one of the only sane ways I've found to cope with the absurdities involved with this experience—maybe I should say one of the only ways to keep *me* sane as I cope with the absurdities.

I think you know what I mean. How else *can* you respond when you find yourself in a crowded line sandwiched between two very, very pregnant women? Explaining to your boss that you're having to miss work to have a hystersalp—, hystersalping—, hystersa—, a tube test? Thinking up a believable explanation for a policeman as you speed your husband's semen analysis sample to the doctor ("What's in the jar, lady?")? Squelching an urge to stomp on the little church lady's toes who's asking you, "Dear, don't you like children?"

Coping. What does it really mean, anyway? "You sure are coping well," one friend casually remarked as I mentioned my morning spent in the doctor's office. *I am?* I thought. *You should have seen me yesterday.* The day before, two of my favorite friends both had their first babies. One after a miscarriage, the other after eight years of infertility. I did wonderfully, even to the extent of going to the hospital. And I knew I was past a very important hurdle because I was truly happy for them . . . until almost imperceptibly, as I stood gazing through the nursery's window talking of inches and pounds and labor and joy, I realized I wasn't focusing on my friends and their happiness anymore, as much as I tried. Instead, I was focusing on the sudden turmoil going on inside me. Quickly I had made my excuses and rushed outside into the fresh air.

Did I cope well? Good question. Depends on your definition of "cope." *Webster's New Collegiate Dictionary* defines it: "to maintain a contest or combat usually on even terms or with success."

". . . on even terms or with success." Yes, that is exactly what coping is for us in this fertility crisis. We are coping when we find ourselves, not sinking, but holding our heads above water—even pulling ourselves up out of the waves that push and shove us daily. To cope, then, *is* to overcome, but not necessarily. Sometimes—most of the time—it's just to hold your own. Let's, then, talk about ways to do either/or.

One of the first ways we realize that we are coping with this crisis is when we understand that the emotions we feel *will pass.* And that they are not wrong.

I'm still learning that truth, to this very moment. Two weeks ago several notable things happened to me at the same time. I finished writing the chapter on emotions for this book—learning and feeling a lot in the process; I found out that our latest attempt at pregnancy had been futile; *and* I received the first copy of my first book—*my very first book.*

A normal writer would have been doing cartwheels over that last event. But I didn't. I sat and stared at that book with my name on it, waiting to feel that thrill, demanding myself to be ecstatic just as I had always pictured myself being at that moment. Oh, I felt good—but not ecstatic. So I became mad, frustrated, upset at myself. And worried. What was wrong with me? Why wasn't I feeling the right feelings? A dense blue fog had lowered over me and would not go away. It wasn't that it hadn't happened before. It had. And it had passed. But my personal expectations overshadowed everything. I should be doing those cartwheels, I told myself, and something must be terribly, permanently wrong because I wasn't. I worried that I wouldn't write the rest of this book; I worried that I would never be able to enjoy anything again; I worried that I'd go through life like a cartoon character with my little blue fog floating over me forever—and on and on the way worry goes.

That was Thursday. On Sunday, I was reading my book and suddenly that thrill *rushed* over me. Instantly, the blue fog lifted, as it had always done before. And I saw everything clearly, sharply. I realized I had expected too much of myself with so many emotional things going on, and vowed to remember that for the next blue fog attack. And I went back, joyfully, to my reading.

I believe that is coping. Awareness is a major part of the effort. As one woman has come to understand her own situation:

> There are many times when I feel just rotten. . . . During those times I know not to make any drastic decisions. I let myself feel the intensity; there is nothing wrong with it. In fact, I have found that there is something right about feeling it, and then letting it move through me, because it always brings me to a more clear understanding of what I want and what my next step should be.[1]

Coping begins, I believe, when we start to focus less on "Why am I having trouble with my fertility?" and more on "How do I handle it?" You might come to a moment when you feel you've had enough—a moment when you realize that there's nothing to be ashamed of, that you've done nothing you cannot talk about and handle, and that there is something very unhealthy about denying, hiding a fact of life you're going through. An editorial in a RESOLVE newsletter summed up the point beautifully in its title alone: " 'Coming out of the Closet' (or What Were You Doing in There in the First Place?)."

From that moment, you begin talking to your spouse, your friends, family, yourself, maybe even writing down your thoughts, your reactions. That moment is a good sign. It means you're on your way to coping on "even terms"—allowing your feelings to wash over you and float away, holding your own in deep water, and it means you're on your way to coping "with success"—pulling yourself up out of the deep end to where you can touch bottom.

Such healthy coping in the long run must not be a fragmented thing, although it may begin that way. It should finally flow through every area of life—your marriage, your family, friends, your attitudes, your health—every area that the fertility crisis has touched.

MARRIAGE

Remember how you felt when you were first married, the feeling that you and your love could handle anything? That there was nothing out there big enough to ever come between you? By now, you two have had time to test that feeling many times probably. Life has already thrown you several curves, and you've held on beautifully. Nothing out there *was* big enough to come between you.

And then came infertility . . . and everything seemed different.

Infertility is a force in marriage that is like no other, because it does not come as much from "out there" as from "in here." It is not so much an outer force, as an inner one that nibbles away at areas hard to talk about: your individual self-image, your sexuality, your sexual relationship, your emotional well-being, your ways of responding to crisis—every area of your marriage from the inside out. And though you may want to cope with this crisis through a united front, it just may not be possible at first. Because so many deeply personal issues are involved, you will more than likely find that you are coping in different ways and at different times than your spouse. And that can begin your drift apart.

My husband and I are a textbook case of a couple who responds to life in diametrically opposite ways. I'm a questioner; he's a believer. I'm a go-getter; he's an accepter. In past problems, after learning the hard way that neither way of coping is wrong, we learned to steer around this difference (usually) and work *with* it somehow toward solutions. But infertility was not the normal problem. And we in essence went our separate ways, coping-wise. And it hurt.

But in doing so, we again became a textbook sort of case— we became like most couples who go through infertility: I talked incessantly; he kept it all in. Does that sound familiar? The average couple will go through a scenario something like this:

He will cope by keeping it to himself and focusing on her. . . . She will cope by expressing over and over how awful and unfair and frustrating everything is. . . . She pushes more and more; he retreats more and more. . . . He feels overwhelmed by her need because he feels powerless to take away the pain; she feels abandoned when she needs him the most. . . .

And the scene goes on night after night after night.

Some men may *not* feel the crisis anywhere as personally as their wives. As we've explored, possible infertility is harder on the wife because of our culture's female role conditioning. His seems to be a broader future "life image," filled with many more things than parenting compared to her picture of "many more things *after* parenting." But a woman cannot assume from her husband's silence that he isn't hurting too. She could be grieving for two. Listen to how one male client of Dr. Mahlstedt expressed it:

> My wife is upset about different parts of the experience with infertility than I am. She feels like a failure . . . crying so much of the time. I hate going through all of this too, but I am most upset over what it is doing to her. . . . As a result, when I do feel like crying . . . I don't because I'm afraid my crying would make her feel worse. And she believes I'm not upset. I'm playing a game, and we are both losing.[2]

After months or years of this sort of tension, even a marriage made in heaven will feel the strain. The scenario, though, is not always "wife talking/husband clamming-up." An indirect channeling of anger can easily surface at home. Little things you've always been able to handle with ease become big issues. And you may end up spending your time and energy blowing up over other matters when it's really infertility you're angry at and should be coping with.

The issue is so, so personal. You cannot help but look at your marriage differently as you look at yourself differently. And as the crisis forces a spotlight on your marital relationship, the easiest thing to do is to keep dodging the light. But you can't. Boston psychiatrist Miriam Mazor sees the point clearly: "Infertility makes couples take a harder look at each other. . . . They begin to assess the marriage at a stage when other couples are too busy with child care to do so."[3] The health of your relationship must stand the glare of that spotlight and must keep standing the glare for the whole infertility crisis—however extended that may be.

What's the answer, then?

Communication.

But how can there be any communication if one of us is doing all the talking and the other is doing all the ignoring? What can we do about that? Psychotherapist Merle Bombardieri has thought up one very hopeful, helpful thing you as a couple can do, a simple idea that can begin that pivotal communication. She calls it "The Twenty-Minute Rule." Her idea is for you to set a timer for twenty minutes or so and then limit each night's discussion to just that amount of time. The result should be that the wife will talk, but she'll crystallize what she wants to say into the small amount of time, and the husband will listen because he knows he doesn't have to listen all night. As Bombardieri puts it, "Less is more in this instance."[4] And surprisingly enough, when the wife talks less, the husband may talk more. In fact, one good idea is for the wife to ask her husband pointedly, "What's it like for you?" and then listen quietly. The only exception to this rule would be, of course, an awful day of bad medical news or another family pregnancy. But for the day-in, day-out infertility grind, this rule can work wonders.

And communication can begin. There is a trick to communication, however. The trick is to listen without criticism and advice, and with acceptance and understanding. It's hard to assimilate such a serious life situation. Even if you decided this very second to change, your coping patterns will be slow in transition. And you must know that about both you and your marriage partner. But you as partners must also remember that, as psychologists Barbara Harvey and Allen Harvey explain, "Solutions will come only with successive confrontations in recurring periods of examination. But the process of coping is speeded up if communication between partners is open and forthright."[5]

As you talk, you'll find yourselves growing together. Slowly you'll grasp what's happening to you. To yourself and your spouse. And you may begin thinking of ways to cope together. The husband might decide to be with his wife through as much of her part of the medical work-up as possible. You may decide together that there are ways to soften the tension of temperature charts, the husband keeping the chart or picking between the two or three pivotal nights, for instance. Maybe you can explore other ways to share, working toward coping in a healthy, partnership way.

Sometimes, though, it takes more than just "one-on-one" talking to really feel you are "on even terms or with success" with this layer of the crisis. What you may need to do is bounce your ideas off other couples, hearing that you are normal, hearing how they are responding. Many, many couples cannot get past their own denial without sharing with other couples going through the same thing. You might want to share with another couple who is going through the same crisis, or you might want to seek out a group. Your specialist should know of such groups. RESOLVE, the national infertility organization, certianly offers you that, now having groups across the country. (They also offer a hotline for you to call, a continually expanding list of infertility literature, a newsletter full of medical updates, helpful information, encouraging articles and possible contacts you can make in your area. See Appendix.)

Sound hard? Maybe it is. But having a healthy marital relationship calls for effort, even without being pulled down by a life crisis such as infertility. Infertility is a *shared* problem. It must be. Whose medical problem it is matters not. You are facing the crisis as a couple, and both of you will have problems to work through. And if you already have a trusting, mutually supportive relationship, you'll find this concept easier to comprehend. The battle must be from that united front, not a *You vs. Me vs. The Problem*, but a *You* and *Me vs. The Problem*.

My husband and I realized we were at this point after several years of fertility testing. We had been on that mind-numbing "normal" infertility treadmill forever, it seemed, before we finally found one questionable problem. Now we could easily have the extra burden of thinking that maybe, just maybe, if we had married someone else we would have been parents by now. But amazingly enough, the thought did not occur to either of us for quite some time after that. It was a revelation that came up quite casually as we were talking and cruising down the highway. We looked at each other a little strangely and sort of smiled. And then there was a silence—in which we both knew that such a thought was not even thinkable, not worthy of words. Because we knew, without words, that we valued our relationship above children. And that's the way marriage was meant to be.

Ours is a society that gives us many role models for our future parenting, but few for a future marital relationship separate from parenting. So, it's easy to feel confused about it all. But what is the reason for being married? Would we answer, "To have children?" Well, I suppose we can't rule out the possibility that some people get married exclusively for that reason. But in our modern society, the idea sounds not only manipulative, but self-defeating. A marriage is first and last a relationship of two, a nurturing of each other, a sacred union—if we believe our marriage vows. To believe that a child is the only result of a healthy marriage is to miss the value and bonding of marriage.

So maybe we should stop and ask ourselves *why* we want to parent. To carry on the family name? To have someone to love? To live through our offspring? To be like "everyone else?" Yes, a child is of value. But isn't our marriage partner of much more value? Yes, parenting is probably what we've always pictured we'd be doing together in the future, but isn't the picture of "together" the most important of all? And are we so rigid that we can't change that picture if we must? The time is ripe for exploring such questions honestly, alone and together.

Such a united front may not feel so natural right now. Dr. Mazor is right. We're scrutinizing our marriage much more closely and much more quickly than our "child-filled friends." We may worry that it won't stand the once-over. Many marriages don't. We're fighting a lot of battles, putting out a lot of fires on lots of fronts. So, our coping may have to be first on a personal level.

One reason for that is the fact that while we're looking at each other, we're also looking within ourselves. Our vision of our personal sexuality cannot help but be a little marred. Our feelings about our maleness and femaleness is integral to our innate understanding and acceptance of ourselves, but the only time we might ever question those feelings is when we can't have a child—which points out how infertility and sexuality are intertwined. And none of us are immune to thinking that somehow our sexuality is at fault. As one woman put it, "At this point even a miscarriage would represent progress because then I'd know I could conceive. I feel a deep and profound sense of failure as a woman."[6] Another had the erroneous idea that her husband's low sperm count must be a sign of his lack of interest in her. "If only I was a more desirable woman, my husband wouldn't have this problem."[7]

The only way to cope with this problem is to ask yourselves what does it mean to be a man or a woman? Do you prove your sexuality by pointing to offspring? Some might, but what would that have to do with what and who they *are?* Sexuality is how a person thinks and feels about being the sex he or she is. It is not sensuality and it is not sexual fertility. It has nothing to do with sexual attractiveness or sexual performance. Past the conditioning of society we must begin to see ourselves in our own light—and reevaluate, if need be.

This of course, brings up another marital stress point—the sexual relationship. The havoc that infertility wreaks with a couple's sexual relationship is positively criminal and, in a very painful way, becomes the pivotal worry of most infertile couples. A study of thirty-five infertile women showed that virtually all experienced a destruction of their sex life and a worry that they'd never enjoy sex again.[8]

Your medical work-up will intrude, and keep intruding, no matter what you do for a time. "Mental charting," which goes on even after you burn your charts and toss your thermometer, will still be a potential form of sexual stress. You know too much about your body now not to know when your fertile times are—when *the* nights should be. Many couples talk of feeling burned out. But how else can you feel when it seems you're forced into separating love from sex?

"Getting back to romantic, spontaneous, and pleasureful sex may take a long time, but it can come back," declares Barbara Menning, from her long experience in counseling.[9] The hiatus may last until the grieving is over or until some resolution. But through all this, remember that your spouse still has the need to know he or she is loved and attractive. And the good news is that the thirty-five women in the study above also stated that their marriages were better for the infertility experience and that they now discussed things with their husbands that they wouldn't have otherwise.

Keeping your marriage healthy through this crisis may mean communicating in a new way, in a deeper way than you ever have before. It may mean looking painfully deep into yourself, into your long-held understanding of your own sexuality, your own beliefs about marriage, and your own priority system. And then it may mean listening closely to the one you hold dearest as he or she works through all the painfully deep examinations too. The united front is possible. And surviving the emotional, mental, and physical stress of infertility can forge a marital bond that can face anything—and survive.

COPING WITH FAMILY AND FRIENDS

Does *anyone* understand? That's what we want to ask when we hear such comments as these:

"What do you *do* all day?"

"Can't you get your mind off this infertility for a little while and just enjoy yourself?"

"Why haven't you made vice-president yet, since you don't have any kids?"

"Now, don't take me wrong, dear, but don't you think it's a little selfish not going to the baby shower?"

"Oh, really, it's not as bad as you think it is, you know."

Some can be downright unkind. One woman's high school friend asked her, "Who are you going to hug, a dollar bill?" At Christmas, her mother asked, "Are you going to have a tree?" as if two people were not enough to enjoy common holiday traditions.[10] Another woman was constantly hounded by her mother-in-law to have a child, until she finally blew up and blurted: "Go talk to your son. It's his fault we can't have kids!"[11]

You know as well as I do that telling such people about your problem is no guarantee they'll understand. A friend of mine quipped that at least I didn't have to worry about birth control. Another told me that I wouldn't have to experience the "empty nest" problem in mid-life. And another pointed out all the money we'd save. And *another* reminded me how much harder it was to get back into shape after a pregnancy at my age.

What do you do?! If you're like me, you usually smile, swallow the highly deserved retort, and politely mumble some meaningless response so you can change the subject and make an exit. As much as we'd like it to be, the healthy answer is not to cut ourselves off from the whole baby-producing planet. For our own sake and for the sake of our relationships, we must *talk*. Intellectually, we can understand our situation quickly enough, but our gut-level feeling is a different matter. Talking will make the difference. And the positive reactions of your close friends and family may be just what you need to get you on the road to coping effectively, to healing. As one friend put it,

> I realized our problem, and though I thought I was accepting it, I was actually worried about what everyone else thought. Finally, I told a friend and she reacted with her own anger, and her own frustration—for me! What she did was affirm me—and my feelings. To see my feelings bounced off another made me realize I was okay.

Yet what about those people who don't respond so affirmingly, who make those crude remarks and have all the advice?

RESOLVE founder Barbara Menning asks in response, "Why do infertile people feel they have to endure such painful comments or situations?" "Well," we might answer, "we must be polite," or "Or it wouldn't do any good." Such thinking might just make the situation worse. As Menning goes on:

> If [the couple] keeps their infertility secret or they honestly give up on people by thinking, "They just could not understand," then the infertile couple are unwittingly setting themselves up for one painful encounter after another—or worse, withdrawal into total isolation in an attempt to be safe.[12]

We must realize that people should be made accountable for their remarks. But that can only happen after we've honestly explained what hurts and what helps to the people who really matter to us.

The risk, of course, is that in being open with a fertility problem we'll become objects of pity instead of empathy and understanding. And pity is awful. A friend does not pity. A friend empathizes. Yet empathy is a special quality, one that comes only from identifying with a similar pain. Is that possible for the person who's never been through infertility? Yes, if they care. One RESOLVE member shared how:

> Last week during a walk with a good friend, I was deeply moved when she displayed real empathy for my infertility experience. My friend is . . . a mother [so] her understanding did not spring from attempts to imagine what it would be like not to have a child. Instead, I know that in order to give such invaluable support to me, she drew upon her own experience with grief caused by a painful divorce. . . . I spent some time thinking about just what it means to be empathetic and to give support. Our empathy for another's pain . . . can only come from a willingness to draw upon our own sadness and to realize that what that other person is feeling is essentially the same.[13]

To explain that dynamic to your friends may be exactly what they need to empathize with your feelings. And to hear your closest friends or family respond in a loving manner may be just what *you* need. Such empathy is a lesson you're learning, too, and one that you will be able to use with others who are hurting. Realize, though, that empathy calls for a willingness to draw upon a person's own tragedies, and some may not be able to make that sacrifice for you. In that case, the ball is back in your court, and how you respond to your relative's or friend's inability to cope with your problem is up to you.

"Up to me?!" you might scream. "They're the ones who are being cruel, insensitive, and uninterested!" It truly hurts to open up to someone only to find out they cannot pull you in and give you sustenance and comfort. But as you begin to cope, how you respond is up to you. It must be up to you. When you begin putting the blame on others, you are giving the whole world the power to control you.

Some people are hopeless. Crude old Uncle Homer may never be able to change. And surprisingly, some friends may keep making jokes; others may not have what it takes to em-pathize. Some family members and others in your life may just continue to meddle. One healthy response you might try in this case is to shift the focus from you to the insensitive ques-tioner. For instance, if someone asks you for the umpteenth time if you're ever going to have children, you might answer: "What is it about my not having children that bothers you so much?" Too confrontive? I don't think so. Not if this is a re-curring scene. However you respond, though, you'll know you're coping well when you do not give such people the power to upset you, no matter how insensitive the remark.[14]

Risks or no, then, talking *is* the only avenue to a healthy coping pattern. In Section 1, we mentioned the similarities be-tween the stages of grief in dying and the stages of emotion with infertility. There's one more similarity. Research has shown that widows who had the opportunity to talk repeatedly about their loss and the changes in their life-expectations suf-fered fewer physical illnesses, connecting stress with higher incidence of physical illness.[15] The word "repeatedly" should be underlined, however. By doing nothing more than being available, a friend can help you get through all those emotional stages faster and saner.

Doing that, though, may not be the easiest thing in the world for your friends and family. Why? Because most people who want to be helpful will feel they must *do* something. They feel compelled to reassure you. That's why you hear such remarks as: "I'm sure it will turn out all right" or "I had a friend that had this problem, and she has three kids now." They may also try to diminish the problem: "Oh, it's not as bad you think it is." "All you have to do is relax or take a vacation. It'll come naturally." "Life's not just having kids you know."

All such comments will only give you the feeling that you're overreacting or that you are probably at fault in some way. But in reality, the only thing a friend or relative should *do* is *be*. A friend who knows how to listen with warmth, love, and uncritical understanding can offer you something positively therapeutic. Being there is the important thing—being there, listening, allowing you to work through your own private world of feeling and being and doing. And there is only one way for you to have such a friend. That is to tell those you know that care for you just exactly what you need, remembering that because they care for you they *want* to know how to help. The same openness and communication you need in your marriage you need in other close relationships.

Many couples find this sort of "therapeutic" help in groups. As mentioned before, by offering them a place where they can talk openly about their feelings and find the support they need, RESOLVE and its support group program has done wonders for many, many couples. Groups are not for everyone, but they can be a wonderful support in the truest sense of the word.

Educate your friends to what you're going through. If you can't bring yourself to spill everything to everyone near to you, then hand them a book like this, and ask them to read it. Having people you care about read articles and books on what you're going through is a good idea, even for those you do tell all. You'll be amazed at what a difference it makes for them to know that others feel the same as you do.

"Okay," you might ask, "how do you cope with the people who aren't the hopeless case or the casual acquaintance or the caring friend? You don't have to put up with my Cousin Sadie every Christmas!" For that sort of person, there is anger. No, not aggressive anger—but *assertive anger*, the kind one that takes the initiative to explain in a strong yet respectful manner how such questions hurt you and why. And that you'd appreciate their understanding. To take an assertive position is to feel in control. And believe it or not, it works.[16] Cousin Sadie may act as if her feelings are hurt, but she'll stop the questions—or she may actually begin to sympathize. And if not, then you have every right to isolate yourself from such "friends" and family as much as possible.

Another way assertion is relevent to your situation is the way it can be used to handle how you respond to those situations that can push you emotionally over the limit. When you can articulate what events are emotionally stressful to you, you can make the decision to avoid them. To voice these feelings with your spouse or with your friends not only helps you to be honest in your responses to such situations, but also affirms at the same time your right to honor those emotional needs.

For instance, *baby showers* . . .

There is no reason in the world for you to attend events that you know in advance are potentially emotional dynamite. I have come to terms with baby showers for this reason. I have several logical reasons now for not being pressured into going. Period. I don't make excuses, I just buy a present ahead of time, give it to the person giving the shower, and express regrets I can't get in on the fun. Usually, those involved know of my situation and express understanding regrets that I won't be there. If they don't know why, telling them does no good, I have learned. Either you get pity or a friendly lecture on how you are just terribly self-centered.

To tell you the truth, one of the proudest moments I've had in my coping experience was with my last baby shower invitation. After handing the present to the casual friend giving the shower, I told her I couldn't make it. "Really? Why?" she asked. In the past I would have mumbled out some lame excuse, ducked my head, and left. This time I smiled and said, "I just can't make it. Sorry. Have a lot of fun."

Well, *is* it self-centered not to be able to join in the happiness for another? Being the overly sensitive person I am, for years I castigated myself with every invitation. "*Surely* I'm big enough to handle this!" I'd think. And then a friend made an offhanded remark that set me straight: "Why," she asked "do we believe we should be able to handle everything? What has given us the idea that we must be perfect? We expect too much of ourselves." And there is much truth to that for any infertile couple trying to keep a stiff upper lip through the baby-clad world.

But there's another reason for not going to every baby shower that sprinkles into your life. In a very real sense, I now see *going* as self-centered. Since most of the people at the shower would know about my situation, the focus would not be on the guest of honor, but on me. All eyes would stray to see how I was reacting, how I felt, how I coped. That's not being self-conscious, that's just fact. And it's true even for office parties celebrating someone's baby. Making an appearance, wishing your co-worker well, is enough. The focus, though, may still be on you, whether you like it or not, especially if you work with sensitive people who care for you. Out of the six people in my department, three came by to see how I was after the last baby celebration.

There's one more group we must consider—those people we meet that ask us *the* inevitable killer question. Wise words from a RESOLVE newsletter article say it all:

"No," I said, as a quiet response to a polite and fleeting inquiry. . . . There was no longer a need to justify my existence by explaining all I had gone through. . . . There had been far too many times before when such an innocent display of the social graces had left me devastated. . . . But I had said "no." How can such a tiny word denote such a crucial battle won?

She had asked, "Do you have any children?" And I had simply said, "No."[17]

With family and friends, you have the right to your feelings and you have the right to have them honored. With others, "on even terms and with success" will come only from within you. Those who care for you will understand, but you must be honest and open with them. The risk of opening up *is* real. Through assertiveness and a few good experiences with sharing, though, you'll weather the hurtful times better and better.

HEALTH

For your mental health and your physical health, coping is a must in this crisis, as in any crisis. Stress can play havoc with your whole physical presence. But learning to work with the stress of infertility is possible.

Diffusing stress can be started by meeting the problem head on. We've all heard of the fight or flight syndrome of stress that experts talk about, how such a stress response helped the cave man survive by preparing him to fight or to flee. But the all-over body response that helped that cave man can just about do us in. We can't fight and we can't flee, so we wrack our brains for ways to find logical solutions. And the result is worry, worry, and more worry.

One way to diffuse such stress is to wrestle mentally with the one question we do not want to face. . .

Ask yourself: *What am I worried might happen if we can't overcome our infertility?* Confront that question, examine it, and decide how you'll survive it.

What *could happen?* You might not have your own biological children. Your friendships may be affected. The stress of the struggle could crumble your marriage. You might not be able to cope.

Having looked at the worst, next ask yourself, *What can I not avoid about this crisis?* The only totally uncontrollable possibility is that you might not have your own biological children. Your marriage does *not* have to crumble. Your friendships will not *all* be affected. You *can* cope.

Then ask yourself: *What* can *I control? What are my alternatives?* You can fill in the blanks here: You can adopt; you can try one of the new procedures; you can remain childfree. You can work on your marriage; you can be open with your friends and family; you can choose to do one thing a day toward coping healthily. Doing such a mental exercise gives you more of a sense of control, for you feel you are prepared for anything that can happen. And that's one big mentally healthy step.

Sometimes coping with infertility means knowing when to quit. . . . The "normal" infertile couple, as well as the couple who is continually going through therapy after therapy, can be on the fertility quest for years. If this is where you are, you may feel you'll spend the rest of your life between therapy and examination room, a little grey-haired couple charting your temperature forever. One day, though, you begin to consider that word . . . quitting, and the feeling that you want to get on with living. Coming to that point is also a mentally healthy step. A big one—toward *resolution.*

What does "resolution" mean? It describes an attitude of determination with which people tackle a problem and deal with it. So in a sense you know the word well. But it also means to bring a situation to a conclusion. So both meanings apply to us while we're going through the medical work-up and as our treatments run their course. Such resolutions *can* come through having a child, finding out your infertility is permanent, or deciding to quit. And the feeling is described at the end of Section 1 as a peace, a philosophical acceptance, a renewed energy.

However, for many people, such resolution sometimes seems

impossible. There are types of infertility that don't have conclusive endings. In these types, there can always be one more doctor to see, one more treatment to try. And even if you decide to stop everything, there is always the lingering feeling that you might have done more. Like a chronic illness, this sort of infertility with no conclusive end becomes a life-style you feel you'll live forever. How do we cope during that "forever?" When resolution seems all but impossible?

Psychologist Jeanne Fleming, who has gone through infertility herself, has an answer. In her study on this tension of the fertility crisis, she sees a very relevant connection between what she calls "uncertain" infertility and chronic illness:

> Infertility, when not "cured" by pregnancy or diagnosed as permanent, is by definition a chronic illness. It may be threatening to health or even life; it affects daily life—what you do, think and feel; and it requires ongoing adjustments, medically and emotionally. There are varying levels of hope for recovery or eventual resolution of the medical problems and the feelings.[18]

In her study of the literature on coping with chronic illness, Dr. Fleming found that the focus is not on resolution, but on coping and adaptation. And part of adaptation is "healthy avoidance." In coping with a chronic illness, avoidance is not only helpful but often necessary. And so it is with infertility. Healthy avoidance means it is not only all right but also healthy for you to avoid situations that may bring up emotions that cannot be resolved now. Dr. Fleming does point out that this doesn't mean that feelings should be avoided, because denying or burying feelings doesn't work either. At times those feelings need to be expressed very strongly, as we've mentioned. But she believes that such feelings should be seen as clues that your feelings are too strongly out of control and that the best recourse is to focus in a big way on areas of life that offer you more control, success, and pleasure.

Such healthy avoidance might involve missing some family

rituals that make you feel uncomfortable, not being around couples who have children or who aren't empathetic with your feelings, not going to group outings where the emphasis is on the family.

But lest you wonder if avoidance is just another form of isolation, it isn't. For the infertile couple, such avoidance is not forever chronic. It should exist just long enough to help you cope and adapt with the seemingly "forever" state of your infertility work-up. As your attitudes change and you focus on areas of strength and control, as you begin to cope better and better and move toward your own form of resolution—be it a philosophical acceptance, a daily adaptation, or a mixture of both—you'll be able to cast off this avoidance pattern. Until then, though, this strategy would help you keep careful awareness of your feelings so that you can do what you need to do for yourself, *when* you need to do it.

Another part of such adaptation offers us another healthy coping idea. As you find yourself floundering in the middle of "uncertain" infertility it's easy to wonder if there's any way to handle the situation *now.* If we must live this experience, is there any way to live it productively? to feel whole? to feel healed, mentally and emotionally if not physically? Yes, I think so. Besides the concept of "healthy avoidance," coping with infertility as a chronic illness can offer a special sort of coping as-you-go.

When one friend came to the conclusion that her infertility was not a problem to be solved but a continuous, chronic condition that fluctuated as she lived through it, she began to put her thoughts into a journal:

> As a sufferer I was trapped by my expectation that only when this whole problem was solved would I be well, good again, whole. But that is like a blind man saying he'll wait until he sees again to live productively. The way out is not so much problem-solving, as "healing." And healing has to do with making whole—restoring integrity, rather than finding answers.

What is my goal? Pregnancy, of course. But more—it's to feel whole if I never become pregnant. Not "well," maybe, but "healed," in an emotional sense. . . .

Maybe the best thing is to put your quest for a baby on the back burner for awhile. Take a vacation from it all, at least in a mental sort of way. Relaxation and a little peace of mind may surprise you by coming naturally as you center in on other areas of life like self-esteem, hobbies, and talents, concentrating on feeling whole and seeing life as a whole. Such a break can be nothing but mentally healthy for your pooped psyche.

Then as you are gaining that new perspective, a little self-confidence might lead you to another thought: as unwilling victims in this "crime," maybe you might find something very right in a little righteous anger—in deciding that you just will *not* be a victim. As the same determined woman wrote in another journal entry: "Embrace my problem? Probably never, but if the alternative is to become a victim, then I will. I shall not lend control of my life to this unwelcome, unmerited catastrophe. It will *not* be said of me that a 'failure' defined my life." To mix such a form of resolve with other ways of coping might be just the fuel you need.

The state of your mental health in this crisis cannot be ignored or belittled. Remember that just as a person recuperating from a physical injury is vulnerable to complications, so is a person who is juggling emotional complications of the fertility crisis. Another crisis in your life at this time may wreak havoc with your ability to cope. In a very real, very serious sense, your usual coping patterns may not be able to handle the burden of two crises. Loss of a job, serious illness, death of a loved one—situations that are hard to bear at any time may be too much right now for you to cope with effectively.

Also, the infertile couple can easily begin to think that all their problems are the result of their fertility problem. Dr. Mahlstedt has found this to be true in her counseling with infertile couples. Often she will ask her clients to tell her about things that are happening in their lives and lead them to see they are not related to their infertility problem at all.

So be easy on yourself, and if you need to, go for counseling. Your doctor can be a good source for a competent professional experienced in infertility counseling. Never forget that anyone going through a major life crisis may need professional help.

COPING TIPS

What else can you do? Plenty. Psychotherapist Merle Bombardieri and several RESOLVE members have written some fine articles listing practical, on-target ways in which to cope with the stress of infertility. Most of the following ideas come from their writings on the subject:

1. Set realistic goals. Your ability to cope with the stress of infertility takes time. And a certain amount of stick-to-it-ive-ness.
2. Recognize your own stress signs. Begin monitoring what makes you tense—for instance, your inner voice saying, "A really mature person wouldn't be this upset over not having a baby."
3. Stop feeling rotten about feeling rotten. Something terrible is happening to you, and you're supposed to feel rotten! These are normal responses to infertility and should be recognized as such.
4. Build a bridge back to your family.
5. Remember you can explain how you and your spouse are having trouble having a baby without telling everyone—or anyone—the nitty-gritty details of your medical experience.
6. Give yourself permission to cry, be angry—feel your feelings. If you feel overpowered, though, give yourself a little control over those feelings by fencing them in. Set a limit on them, too. Decide to feel awful, depressed,

angry for thirty minutes a night, if it will help. Then get busy with other things.

7. Do something special for your spouse at least once a week—keep your marriage strong.

8. Allow your spouse to cope in different ways and at different times than you.

9. Be assertive not only with friends but with doctors.

10. Learn as much as you can about your medical problem and work-up.

11. Take a break from charts, thermometers, and treatments, if at all possible.

12. Take up a hobby you're always saying you'd like to.

13. Stop putting off plans for your future and seriously discuss alternatives with your spouse.

14. Keep a journal. You'll be amazed at what you learn when you see your feelings on paper.

15. Start talking back to yourself: When you hear yourself say, "I'll never get pregnant," answer: "I don't really know what will happen, but we're going to a specialist and doing all we can." When you think, "Our sex life is ruined forever," answer: "It's only normal for sex during infertility to be a chore. We have every reason to expect our sexual relationship to be restored when the crisis is over." When you think, "I should have tried to get pregnant five years ago," or "I should be able to make my wife happy," realize you are doing your best.

16. Take care of your health. Besides rest, recreation, and eating right, plenty of exercise actually burns up the substances that your body produces under stress.

17. Try coping with sexual stress through talking about it, through making time for intimate togetherness apart from schedules, or even differentiating between work sex and fun sex.

18. Look into some stress management techniques, such as deep breathing techniques.

19. Learn how to meditate. Concentrate on your spiritual life.

20. As for those family-oriented holidays that we all know to be times of amazing tension, decide to make them *your own*. How? During the holidays, make a point to allow the meaning of the holidays, such as Christmas, Hanukkah, Thanksgiving to sink in. Plan a trip, go out of your way to do something for someone else. Create your own traditions. Don't apologize for joining your family *after* all your nieces and nephews have opened their presents. It's really up to you to understand that the holidays aren't for children. They are celebrated for a larger reason, one that we often miss in the commercial hubbub. Remember that our idyllic picture of the holiday season full of family bliss and happiness is, sad to say, less than reality for most people. So do yourself a favor. Realize that however you're feeling now will pass. Be good to yourself during the holidays, and celebrate their true meaning with the ones you love. Make it special. For you. Apart from outside expectations or pressures.[19]

". . . on even terms or with success." Can we cope? Can we focus less on the "why?" of our infertility and more on the "how do we handle it?" Yes. But it takes effort. And we may not believe at this moment that we have any energy left for it all. But none of us want to allow infertility to ruin our lives. So it's up to us.

Coping isn't asking us to be jump-up-and-down happy with our situation. Coping will probably not even alleviate all the pain and sadness. But what it will do is give us back our lives. And that's no small thing. There really is much that is ours to control. And if our coping attempts do nothing else but teach us that, it's worth the effort.

This is beginning to be a very expensive pastime, *I think as I clutch the flimsy hospital robe around me, checking for exposed parts. I scoot over to the nearest chair in the long, cold hallway and hastily sit down. The hospital walls are a cheery color, not exactly matching my mood. I lock eyes for a moment with an elderly man sitting across from me. He is clutching, too. Embarrassed, we smile and quickly look away.*

How long had it been since I started these trips? *It seemed an eon. But it had been only a handful of months. After about a year of testing and treatment, my gynecologist had asked me to come by for a talk.*

"Want me to go with you?" my husband had gallantly offered as I left for the appointment.

"Naaaw. That's okay," I had said.

"Really, I mean it. If you want me to go, I'll go. Really."

"No, no big deal," I had said.

But it had been a big deal, because my doctor had suggested we do the rest of the testing with a specialist. And he'd even gone so far as setting up the appointment.

"Want me to go along?" my husband had offered once more.

"Yes."

"Really, I mean it. If you want me to go, I'll. . . ."

"I do."

". . . really go. Hmmm? Oh . . . well. Okay. . . ." he had mumbled.

And we had gone, and gone again and again—wandering through the halls of the big hospital together to the specialist, the urologist, the lab technicians, umpteen nurses and receptionists. After awhile, we became fluent in "infertility-ese," using words such as Clomid and

BBT and endometriosis and sperm motility as we went from test to test to test.

And as I got to know the specialist and nurses, I began to ask questions: What's this test? Sperm antibody, you say? Another blood test? Yes, nurse, I'll begin breathing again when you take the needle out. An endometrial biopsy? Won't hurt a bit? It's not "hurting a bit" that bothers me, Doctor, it's "hurting a lot" that has me concerned. . . .

As I adjust my hospital gown, I smile a little, thinking about it all, and sit back in the plastic hospital chair. Then the smile vanishes as I lean my head back against the wall and think about the frustration, the questions, the feeling of helplessness that have trailed along behind these months of tests and treatments and trips to the hospital. All the crazy notions I'd had about what infertility was, all the little fears I had about each test. If somebody had just told me a little more about what to expect, it might have helped. . . . *I think.* Yeah, it would have made it a little easier.

I clutch the robe tighter around me, shivering a little from the chill in the hallway, bladder full and mind numb. My bladder is full as a part of the test I'm about to take, my mind is numb from the thought of having to take another one. Absently, I look around for a magazine, a newspaper, anything to pass the time as I wait for this new test: an ultrasound—one more step in our quest for a baby.

A baby? Is that right? *I frown.* That sounds somehow . . . unfamiliar. *The dream seems to have gotten a little fogged up along the way.*

"Hi." I hear from beside me.

"Oh hi," I mumble as I take in the person behind the friendly greeting and generic robe. Her shape tells me she's here for an ultrasound too, but not for the same reason I am. Are you pregnant? *I want to ask,* or is your bladder in worse shape than mine? *I squelch a laugh, coughing mildly until it's out of my system. I start to share the joke, but decide she might not appreciate it. Besides, I think with a pained expression, laughing right now might be very risky. And I move around a little, trying to get more comfortable.*

"Mrs. Youngblood?"

The woman gets up and walks through the door.

Another door opens.

"Mrs. Stephenson?" The woman glances at the man, then at me. She smiles. I must be the one.

I get up, still clutching, and follow her into a dimly lit room of TV monitors and examination tables.

As she begins to bounce the waves off my stomach in search of ovaries and follicles and eggs, I sigh mentally.

"My, you're doing good," she purrs."I know your bladder being so full is quite uncomfortable for you, but it makes for a great picture for us."

"Not if I float away," I groan.

All is silence as she concentrates, as I endure. She moves the device across me once, twice, around and around—searching. "We try to be as conscientious as possible," she is suddenly saying, "because we know how important it is."

Important? No big deal. It's just another test, *I almost say. Then I suddenly realize how utterly stupid that would sound.* Of course it's important! Why else would I be lying flat on my back in a flimsy robe, in a strange hospital, in a strange city, with a strange woman administering a very expensive test over me? . . . Defense mechanisms on and operating, *I realize.*

"Ah. There," she is saying as I hear the click, click of a picture being taken. "Okay, we're through. You can relieve yourself."

If it were only that easy, *I think, as I rush past the elderly man and down the hall.*

WHAT SHOULD WE KNOW AS WE BEGIN TESTING AND TREATMENT?

The Medical Crisis

It all began so nicely. One day you probably decided that it was time to begin a family. You may have put off starting a family for a while to give yourselves time to get to know each other, begin careers, mature. Or you may have wanted to begin your family from the moment of your vows. But whenever the time had come, you were emotionally prepared and excited, counting the days on the calendar, thinking of the possibilities. After all, you've planned everything else, you might as well plan your child's birthday.

Then a month goes by, then another . . . and another. And soon, you begin to wonder. The months turn into a year, maybe years. And you aren't smiling anymore. You are worrying. Then one day, the braver of you two mentions going to the doctor.

Is this where you are?

For us, the first hurdle was accepting the fact that we might not be normal, might not be like everybody else. We were both healthy, athletic, vigorous individuals who came from large families. Infertility didn't make any sense at all, and life was supposed to make sense.

Just the idea of going to a doctor was hard to swallow. Such a decision is absolutely paralyzing to some people, because, in a sense, making that first appointment means that you have to face the possibility that you *do* have a problem, that you're not normal, not like everybody else. And for many, questioning one's fertility is tangled up in an unholy knot of fears. Denial is a lot easier to handle:

"If we wait just one more month . . ."

"If we try Aunt Susie's suggestions . . ."

"If we go on a trip—a long, relaxing romantic one . . ."

It's easier not to confront the questions for fear of the answers. Questions like: What will the doctor find? What if something awful is wrong? What if he tells us it is hopeless? To some, going for medical help is the same as extinguishing hope.

But the opposite is true. With the current mode of therapies, a couple diagnosed as infertile has about a fifty-fifty chance of becoming parents once the diagnosis has been made . . . And the amazing advances in diagnostic techniques can identify the cause in ninety percent of cases. That figure was forty percent only a decade ago.[1]

WHAT INFERTILITY IS AND WHAT IT IS NOT—THE FACTS

DIAGNOSED AS INFERTILE. Sounds awful, doesn't it? . . . Well, what does the word *infertile* mean? First, it does *not* mean sterile. Sterility means that a person can't conceive under any circumstances. Infertility means that a couple possesses less than the maximum potential for reproduction. It is not a hopeless word, by any means. It means you, and the other ten million in this country, are having trouble conceiving.[2] Infertility as defined by most doctors is the "inability to conceive a pregnancy after a year or more of regular sexual relations without contraceptions, or the inability to carry pregnancies to a live birth."[3]

And contrary to current thought, there is no time in life that you can presume your fertility. As Barbara Menning, founder of RESOLVE, the national infertility organization, explains:

> By . . . definition, fertility can only be known after the fact. Until a conception occurs, a man and woman can think they are fertile, based on family precedents or the odds in general. But they cannot know they are fertile until a conception and live birth have occurred. This is equally true of those who have had previous births. . . . Past fertility tells nothing about present fertility. Fertility is not a life force that may be turned on at will.[4]

We can prevent pregnancy with almost a hundred percent accuracy, but we cannot produce it on demand.

The American Fertility Society puts it this way:

> There are many reasons why a couple may have difficulty getting pregnant. Because of careers and later marriages, more women now choose to conceive later in life, after fertility has naturally declined. New methods of birth control have affected fertility. But individual medical problems in both the female and male are still the leading cause of fertility problems. In only a few couples does infertility remain unexplained.[5]

And there is another factor—the factor of odds. Becoming pregnant is basically a game of odds. Some couples are simply more likely to get pregnant quicker than others. It's been said that if we had three hundred years in which to conceive, almost all couples would become pregnant. But since the average time allotted us is about fifteen years, the odds can be poor. Sometimes it just takes a while for some couples to conceive. In other words, you may be one of the few that takes several years to become pregnant. That might explain what is called the "spontaneous cure rate," which accounts for about five percent of all "infertile" couples each year becoming pregnant by no visible means of medical help.[6]

But knowing that you're part of some sort of univeral dice-rolling is no comfort. One specialist explains fertility this way:

> Think of fertility in these terms: If one were to flip a coin three times in a row, and land tails each time, he might think that on the next flip he would be more likely to land heads than tails. Of course this is not true. Each time the coin is flipped there is a fifty-fifty chance of its landing either heads or tails, regardless of past history.[7]

The average couple has about a twenty percent chance each month of becoming pregnant. Statistics vary, but it's safe to say that about ninety-four percent will become pregnant within the year. For a woman in her late twenties and early thirties, the probability is somewhat lower—ten to fifteen percent each month, with only seventy to eighty-five percent achieving pregnancy within the first year.[8] (Such figures are based on a couple who is probably making love twice a week. That is what a doctor will tell you is the norm—but such assumptions about normalcy, especially when it comes to something as personal as lovemaking, are annoying at best and calculating at worst, too often giving a couple a sort of mark to shoot for, a guide to follow in order to conform. This sort of pressure is one of the reasons infertility is a major life crisis. So keep in mind that only *you* know what is your norm and that such statistics must be understood in your own context.)

Yet, statistics or no, if you suspect a problem, don't put off seeking a doctor's help waiting for your roll of the dice. Just knowing that you are doing something positive will at least alleviate the awesome stress. The trouble may be minor, it may be major, or it may be no trouble at all. But most of the time, it is something a doctor must treat. And that means you must go to the doctor.

As you are contemplating this important decision, and also gaining a good grasp of what infertility is, you should also know what infertility is not:

1. *Infertility is not mainly a women's condition.* Even though most of the testing is done on the woman, and most of

the knowledge is female-related, it's not a predominately female problem. The statistics are forty percent female, forty percent male, and twenty percent a combination factor. (All those poor biblical women come to mind—living with their culture's "curse of barrenness," carrying the whole burden of the "curse," when in reality the "curse" easily may have been with their husbands!)

2. *Infertility is not due to psychological factors, as a rule.* Does stress cause infertility? That's what we hear sometimes, especially when a physical cause is not diagnosed quickly. However, the fact that infertility causes stress, a situation that's ludicrously obvious for anyone experiencing it, is now a widely accepted fact in medical and psychological circles. Leading infertility specialist Dr. Joseph Bellina, in his book *You Can Have a Baby,* attests to this acceptance by giving the "condition" a medical name—"conception stress syndrome."[9]

   Even though stress, in reality, cannot be totally ruled out as a contributing infertility factor (a woman *can* stop ovulating under extreme stress, for instance), the idea of infertility being "all in your head" is essentially a gross misconception, and couples are done a great disservice when told such. As stated earlier, a physical problem is found in ninety percent of all cases thoroughly tested by qualified doctors. The remaining ten percent, the "normal" infertile couples, may have problems that just cannot be diagnosed with the current technology.

3. *Infertility is not incurable.* As stated before, fifty percent of couples who begin an adequate infertility medical workup will respond to treatment and become pregnant. Compare this to the "spontaneous cure rate" of only five percent in couples who have not conceived after a year.

4. *Infertility is not a sexual disorder.* Except for a very small minority of cases, infertility has nothing to do with the ability to perform sexually. This is another of those myths that can only do a disservice to the couple, even becoming a self-fulfilling prophecy.[10] There is a difference between

making love and procreating, and the difference is between your ears and in your heart. And much care should be taken to keep this intimate, special part of your life from being affected by the threat and the fears of infertility.

5. *Infertility is not a curse from God, and it is not wrong to pursue modern medicine's help in having a child.* Infertility is a medical problem, *not* a spiritual one. A few "religious" people (probably ones who have children and/or grandchildren themselves) may claim you'll be "blessed" when you're supposed to, and that your duty is to wait patiently for that blessing and then accept your lot if it doesn't come. There is nothing "spiritual" about this mentality at all. In fact, it's downright cruel. It's the same sort of mentality that would have you ignore the healing miracles that modern medicine can perform now in hopes—in almost a *demand*—that you be singled out for a special supernatural healing. But there's not much difference between fighting an infection, which the vast majority of us would do automatically, and fighting infertility.

Of course, there may be some aspects of infertility treatment that might trouble some people of faith. To take a semen analysis, a specimen must be obtained, and what a man must do to obtain that specimen might not set well with him, especially if he is from a Catholic background. (Specialists can offer alternatives for such people, although they are not as effective.) And some of the more advanced procedures do get into grey areas for anyone with strong ethical and spiritual standards. (Discussed in Section 4.)

Overall, though, an infertility battle should be viewed like a battle against any other medical problem. The mentality that sees it otherwise is another example of the unusual societal attitudes that engulf the infertility issue.

6. *Infertility is not affected by adoption, oysters, vitamin E, or normal exercise.* You've heard as many home remedies as I have, and the interesting part is that all of them have a

ring of truth. You do know people who've become pregnant after adopting; you do know someone who swears by their vitamins or swore off their running and conceived. And such stories give you hope that something, *something* you do or don't do could make *the* difference.

But there is little to substantiate most of these ideas. Science *has* shown that some women who habitually run *very* long distances (thirty to forty plus miles a week) *can* cease ovulating or experience disrupted cycles.[11] But marathon runners do conceive without quitting their grueling regimen. And no one would consider marathon running normal exercise.

And couples who've adopted *are* surprised with conception after a long period of infertility. But remember the five percent spontaneous cure rate and the game of fertility odds. Long-term studies by Dr. Emmett Lamb on infertile couples who adopted show no significant effect of adoption on subsequent infertility. As one doctor put it, adoption does not improve diseased tubes or reduce the ravages of endometriosis. If there is any credence at all to the idea, it might be in the lessening of tension for the random woman whose anxiety affects her ovulation. But, basically, the five percent spontaneous cure rate— the game of odds—makes more sense.[12]

As for vitamins and food cures, the verdict may never be in, so placing your hope in them would be unwise. And, sometimes, it could also prove unhealthy if you overdo it. The best advice is to try them if you like, but bounce the idea off your doctor first before making them a part of your daily regimen in case they might react against any prescribed medicine. And then take them, usually, with more than "a grain of salt."

CHOOSING A MEDICAL PARTNER

How long, then, should you wait before seeing a doctor?
A year? That's what the experts suggest. Some even feel a

two-year wait is warranted. After about a year, you probably would be wise to consider medical help. There are several exceptions to that arbitrary, somewhat clinical rule:

• If you find that the tension and the anxiety are taking over your life, you are justified in starting a medical checkup earlier. If your marriage is becoming strained, if you are preoccupied with when to make love during the month for best pregnancy chances, if you begin thinking of intercourse as a necessary act instead of an expression of love, if you are racked with worries about what might be wrong and even beginning to argue about whose fault it might be, you should definitely begin a work-up as soon as possible.

The idea of infertility usually creeps into a couple's awareness gradually. Some couples may need to take time just to face the idea that they indeed might be infertile. The role of denial is very, very strong—strong enough to affect more than your fertility. Quietly, slowly, the denial can begin to affect your marriage, manifesting itself in strange ways. As one woman shares:

> If we used contraceptives, there was no chance for a pregnancy, and consequently there could be no infertility problem. Or, even surer, if we did not have intercourse, we certainly did not have an infertility problem. And surest of all, if we got a divorce, we clearly had no problem. It became almost easier for us to contemplate divorce than to face the fact of infertility.[13]

To do something . . . to take the initiative . . . to get the questions out where you can handle them can be an enormous relief. Many doctors tell of cases in which their infertility patients became pregnant right after the first visit, attributing it to lessening tensions. And there may be some truth in that.

So when should you begin a medical work-up? First and foremost, as soon as you feel the need to. Your individual needs can never be charted in a graph or described in statistical form.

- Anyone over thirty should consider consulting a doctor after only six months of trying. A woman is at her peak fertility-wise in her mid-twenties, and it gradually tapers up to thirty. Then fertility begins a rapid decline. Male fertility is also at its peak in the twenties, then declines slowly until forty. So time becomes a very real factor.
- Any person who has any sort of fertility-related problem or illness. That would include a woman who has a continually erratic monthly cycle, or who has stopped having a cycle for long periods of time, or has a history of pelvic infections or endometriosis. And it would also include men who've had adult mumps or have any unusual physical situation such as an undescended testicle.[14]
- Although birth control pills haven't been linked to infertility, many women have automatically taken them at one time or another because we believed pregnancy was a foregone conclusion without them. But the birth control pill's regularity can mask problems we are unaware of. Normally, ovulation may not resume until three months after stopping the "Pill". Taking that fact into consideration, if you've been using the "Pill" then discover you haven't conceived after several months off it, you might consider seeking help early.[15]

Well, how *do* you pick a doctor? Should you go to an infertility specialist from the beginning?

Your first reaction may be to see your family doctor, or more probably your gynecologist. Your family doctor can do some of the early testing, such as blood work and semen analysis. Your gynecologist will most surely have some experience in dealing with infertile patients, but whether he has the expertise to take you very far with the testing is another matter. Most gynecologists had a small amount of training in infertility as part of their specialization work. And there are gynecologists who have done some advanced study in infertility, making it an extra interest of theirs. These doctors can offer you many of the simpler testing and treatments, such as Basal Body Temperature charting, post-coital tests, basic blood work, etc. Many of them will also know when you should go to an infertility specialist and will wisely counsel you to do so, even going so far as setting up your appointment for you. That would be the ideal.

What may be *real*, though, is the obstetrician/gynecologist who says he is trained in the treatment of infertile patients and then may tell you there's nothing to worry about. "Just relax." "Take it easy." "You're young and healthy." "These things take time." Alarm bells should be going off in your head when you hear these sorts of comments. At best, he's not taking you and your anxiety seriously; at worst, he doesn't know much about infertility and will waste your time and money if you keep going to him.

And at the *very* worst, he may even make mistakes that will cost you more than time or money. Our loyalty to our doctors is so strong that most of us will trustingly hang in there, never questioning . . . which is exactly what I did. But after several years of tests and treatment by my gynecologist, I was forced to change doctors. Not because I realized it was time to look elsewhere, but because we moved. We had been through every test, every treatment he knew to give—one being a blood test to check on antibodies, which he had routinely sent to a hometown lab. The test came back negative just as all the others had been. We left town with an abnormally-full file stuffed with nothing but normal tests.

After I spent several months with a new gynecologist in our new town, this astute, concerned doctor referred me to a nearby infertility specialist who took one look at my file, pulled that certain blood test from it, and asked where the lab work had been done. As it turned out, in the specialist's opinion the test needed a special sort of lab work. We took the test again, sent it to a special lab in New York—and the test came back positive. After four years, we had finally found something wrong.

Could we have acquired this problem since the first test? If not, would our lives be different if we had known this problem earlier? I do know that if we had not moved, I would probably have never gone to a specialist, and probably would have never known the problem. I hate to think how many couples accept the first diagnosis, or the absence of diagnosis, out of blind loyalty or fear of taking responsibility for their own situation. Too often we operate on a notion that doctors are above questioning. Not until we realize they must be partners in the search and treatment, and not gods to rely on, will the situation change.

So much is happening in the infertility field that your doctor would have to be quite interested in infertility to keep up with the new advances and new methods and with what methods are now out-of-date. In his book *How to Get Pregnant*, Sherman J. Silber tells of a couple who were the victims of such outmoded advice:

> I once had a patient who had been trying unsuccessfully to impregnate his wife for two years. His previous urologist was not particularly interested in infertility. . . . When the report came back from the lab showing a relatively low sperm count . . . the doctor placed the patient on thyroid supplements—a therapy with no scientific basis, routinely used years ago. No attention was paid to a more likely factor, the varicose vein in his left testicle, which the doctor had not noticed.[16]

The patient was feeling hyperirritability caused by the excess thyroid when he came to see Dr. Silber. Silber did a very simple procedure that increased the man's sperm count to normal levels. The man's irritability vanished when he stopped taking the thyroid pills, and three months later the couple was pregnant.

So there are some very good arguments for seeing the infertility specialist from the beginning, if it is at all possible. The infertility specialist is too often thought of as a consultant for last ditch efforts. That's quite an erroneous idea, for in reality, they would rather work with you from the start, thereby having control over all your testing and therapies.

Because infertility is one of the very few medical disorders that is truly a couple's problem, the specialist will usually prefer to see you as a couple, at least in the beginning. Both of you need to be prepared to undergo testing and examination, because the infertility work-up is not complete without study of both partners.

WHAT EXACTLY IS AN INFERTILITY SPECIALIST?

The specialist is different than your gynecologist in the sense that infertility specialists have decided to make infertility a subspecialty and probably have had additional training in such areas as endocrinology, urology, and reproductive physiology. They probably do not take any obstetric patients. They are almost always affiliated with a teaching hospital or infertility clinic, which puts them close to all resources available for uncovering and treating your problem. Usually, they are on the cutting edge of new techniques and methods. And by being affiliated with an outstanding hospital, they are also afforded the ability to consult other doctors, such as a urologist for the man, if further work is required.[17]

More medical specialties are being created that deal with very narrow areas of infertility. "Andrology" is a new subspecialty of urology dealing with male infertility. And some internists make "reproductive endocrinology," the study of hormones, their primary focus. Also, many teaching hospitals and medical centers are looking into the team approach to infertility. The team would include a gynecologist specializing in infertility, an endocrinologist, an urologist, a pathologist, a psychiatrist, specially trained nurses, social workers, and counselors. As you can see, the medical world is certainly responding to this new medical need.[18]

How do you find these specialists? Ideally, your gynecologist will refer you to the nearest one. But you can also contact two very reliable sources: The American Fertility Society, the national medical organization that is concerned with infertility, lists around five thousand gynecologists interested in infertility; and RESOLVE, the national nonprofit infertility organization which offers every kind of help an infertile couple might want or need, lists over nine hundred specialists and even groups them geographically for you. (See Appendix.) It is no exaggeration to say that the expertise of an infertility specialist can save you years in your struggle, and these organizations are ready and willing to help you find that special person who can help.

WHAT SHOULD YOU EXPECT FROM ANY DOCTOR THAT YOU SEE?

- Your doctor should treat you with sensitivity and concern.
  When my husband went to our family doctor to take that first semen analysis, he waited in a full waiting room for an hour. Then when he was finally called up to the desk, the nurse handed him a little jar, told him the doctor would be back soon, and, in a voice loud enough for the whole waiting room to hear, recited the doctor's directions:
  "Take this bottle, go into the bathroom, and masturbate." Needless to say, it took a while for him to produce the specimen.
  The sensitive doctor will treat you with kindness and awareness, and will never seem to be in a hurry. After an examination, if you'd rather be fully clothed to discuss your tests and treatment, tell him so. If there is a morning that he doesn't see his OB (obstetric) patients, ask him to schedule you then. Waiting in a room filled with pregnant women doesn't do much for your state of mind, much less your blood pressure. Your doctor should be attentive to your concerns and stress.
- Your doctor should respect your intelligence, treating you like an adult.
  One doctor called me "kiddo" and smiled paternally and patronizingly at my questions. Then he told me I shouldn't worry my pretty little head over all of it, and suggested I just trust him to do what's best. (That one I did change. Finally.) You should expect your doctor to explain things

in language you can understand. When we must play the role of patient we seem to think we should be able to understand medical terminology or else just not understand, when in reality we have the intelligence to understand what is going on and the right to know and understand. As Barbara Menning of RESOLVE, herself a registered nurse, points out,

> . . . [A] person should try to become familiar with his or her body and its functions, but beyond that, it is the responsibility of the doctor or nurse to explain and interpret words to the level of the patient's understanding. The patient who is in a state of high anxiety or emotional stress hears and perceives selectively and may even have a partial or total memory lapse about things said in such a state. Therefore, the doctor should repeat important points several times. . . . What the doctor says is only half the communication. What the patient hears and understands is the other half.[19]

• Your doctor should have some sort of training in infertility, and should be able to explain it to you.

  This holds true for both the gynecologist and the infertility specialist. The infertility field is an ever-changing one. Your doctor should be continually updating his or her knowledge.

• He or she should inspire confidence, and you should feel comfortable with him or her. Again, you are searching for a partner to work with, not a god to rely on.

Another aspect of the infertility search is one we'd rather all ignore. Money. How much does all this cost? The answer can be pretty awful, especially if you don't have good insurance. And that's enough reason to investigate your insurance status before you jump on the infertility-go-'round, because even that twenty to thirty percent uncovered by insurance can mount up. Depending on the problem, on the length of the work-up, and on the level of complex treatment, exploring your fertility can cost you anywhere from $8 for a blood test to $30,000 and up for five to six in vitro fertilization attempts.

Some couples will only have to go through the first several tests to find out what to do. But the most truly frustrated group are those that fall into the ten percent of unexplained infertility, the so-called "normal" infertile couples. For years, we were part of this group, being tested and tested and tested until it became a game of elimination, not what was wrong but what wasn't wrong. And the bills kept coming. One couple tells of spending four years and $15,000 trying to conceive—four years of tests, antibiotic treatment, fertility drug therapies, and a trip from their home in New York to a Virginia infertility clinic. "In retrospect," one of them said, "it seems amazing, but we never really thought about the money."[20]

And that's the catch. Most infertile couples are so over-whelmed with the desire for children, they don't even consider the costs. And if they aren't careful, their quest for that baby can cause them to be susceptible to expensive, controversial procedures or even common quackery. As Dr. Joseph Bellina puts it, "Infertile couples are among the most desperate people in America. If I said to such a couple, 'I want to treat you by taking off your right leg and sewing it to your left eye,' they'd ask, 'when?' "[21] The best way to insulate yourself from such extra problems is knowledge. Know what the tests and pro-cedures are and what they do. Ask questions and get answers.

Yet don't let fear of the cost stop you from considering an infertility specialist. They may charge up to five times as much an hour as a regular doctor, but you may wind up saving fifty times that amount through a quicker and more on-target di-agnosis and treatment.

It's a big step—deciding to see a doctor. But the best thing about the decision is that you can feel somewhat in control of an otherwise out-of-control dilemma. To be in control, though, means to go in with your eyes open. And that means you must keep in mind that as a science, infertility is in its infancy. Amaz-ing things are being accomplished, but most of it is still a try-

and-see sort of effort. As one specialist explained it to me, there are no absolutes in infertility. Everything is relative. Even the tests and therapies considered most reliable have their small question marks attached.

With that in mind, the best you can do for yourselves is to take that step. Then with a healthy mix of reality and hope, set a timetable, understand the procedures, feel confident in your doctor partner, and then feel good that you are doing all you can—together.

THE MEDICAL WORK-UP—THE SIMPLE PROCEDURES

BASIC TESTING AND TREATMENT

"Well, Mr. and Mrs. So-and-So, first thing I want you to do is not worry. You see, I have your infertility work-up all planned out. Yes, yes. It's all right here. We'll start with a simple *semen analysis* for you, Mr. So-and-So. That will entail viewing your sperm's *motility, morphology, viability, viscosity,* and of course, their ever important *agglutination.*

"Then we'll begin with you, Mrs. So-and-So. First, we'll study your *ovulatory cycle,* using a *basal body temperature chart* then proceed right into studying your hormones. *Hormones,* you know: *estrogen, progesterone, FSH, LH, testosterone* and *prolactin* levels. Then a few blood tests, *sperm antibody,* for instance, would be in order.

"Hmmm, I suppose *Clomid therapy* would be called for at this point, coupled with monthly *post-coital* tests. What? Oh, Clomid's nothing really. A mild fertility pill. Then . . . what? Yes, yes, mild, very mild fertility pill. I'll probably want us to take an *endometrial biopsy* (won't hurt a bit) followed closely behind with the always revealing *hysterosalpingogram* (fallopian tubes, you know).

"And then if it seems warranted, we'll schedule a *laparoscopy.* Just to see if you have *endometriosis,* you know—By the way, you *are* covered by insurance, I assume? It's a surgical procedure, you see. Yes? Good, good—and if we find nothing there, well, I'll probably want you to begin thinking about *AIH*. Yes, *AIH: artificial insemination by husband*. After that we'll have to consider *AID*, yes—*by donor*—or maybe *Pergonal* treatment. What? Oh, sure, some people *do* have quintuplets with Pergonal, but very few. Very few.

"Well now, any questions? I'm glad we've had this little talk. We'll begin tomorrow morning."

Did that make your head spin? If your doctor plunked the whole infertility treatment schedule into your lap on the first visit, that's about what it would sound like, some sort of secret language decipherable only by someone who'd swallowed a medical textbook. You'd probably be sitting there, nodding your head, dazed-eyed, listening yet not hearing a word.

Thankfully, you're not given the whole picture at first. The doctors guide you along, little by little, explaining as they go. Infertility treatment is a sort of follow-the-dots work that can almost be plotted. Yet, if you are like I was at the beginning, you don't want to know every little medical term, every scientific reason for what you'll be going through. You just want the doctor to fix it, no matter what it is. You want to thank him, pay your bill, and have your baby.

For some of the couples who consult a doctor, a test or two or a little knowledge about timing will be all they need to do. But most couples will go through the line of tests and treatment and become quite intimate with some of those foreign-looking words. Your doctor will probably attempt explanation of what he has in mind, and he may do it well enough that you gain a certain understanding of what is happening. But there is no way you can grasp it all from a 5- or 10-minute talk. And you may be reluctant to ask him to repeat everything until you do understand.

Still, you deserve—no, you *need*—to know all there is to know about what you're going through. As I've pointed out before, it's your body and your time and your money. You need to have a good grasp of what's standard for the infertility medical work-up. Being an informed patient is your best hedge against mistakes or problems or inadvertent omissions. It's not unusual to hear of a couple who has gone through years of therapies at huge emotional—not to mention financial—cost only to find out that the doctor omitted a basic test at the beginning that would have identified the problem.

And, you need to know the basics because like most infertile couples you will be tempted to try anything suggested. A friend hands you a newspaper clipping that suggests multi-doses of vitamin B6 as an infertility cure. You stumble across an article that suggests drinking cough syrup to thin problem cervical mucus. Such information will consistently float by you, and you'll probably think seriously about these ideas. Even your doctor might make suggestions. One doctor, for instance, off-handedly suggested that a couple try eating oysters—lots of oysters, in an attempt to improve hormonal levels. And they not only did it, they did it with enthusiasm.

Some of the ideas you hear may have credence and some may be harmless, but others, such as the megadoses of vitamin B6, can actually harm you. Your doctor wants you to conceive almost as much as you do, and he may suggest such things before he gives up and advises you to see a specialist. He will also know which ones can harm you, so you should consult him if you decide to try some of the ideas in your personal pile of information. But only *you* should make the decisions—along with the doctor's medical advice—about what to try. Having a good grasp of the basics of the infertility medical work-up will help arm you with as much knowledge as possible for those decisions.

"But how can anyone understand all that weird-sounding medical jibberish?" I can almost hear you wondering. Believe it or not, all the procedures listed in the monologue at the beginning of this chapter can be understood by any of us. And even though you may not have to experience all of them first hand, you need to know about them. And that's what this section will do—give you a brief, layman's overview of what you can expect once you begin your infertility search.

But even though the order and basic tests *are* simple enough to explain, detailed explanations of each test and each possible problem can—and do—fill books. And such medical-related books are crammed with information you'll want to know. Miscarriage, for instance, is a form of specific infertility that many women must endure and need to know about. The same goes for DES exposure, t-mycoplasma infection, ectopic pregnancies, and other infertility situations that I cannot cover here. Much of what this book tackles will be pertinent to those of you who experience these problems, but I urge you to seek further specific medical information about such conditions as well.

So, although I can't cover every term and condition infertility encompasses, I *can* urge you once again to check some of the fine articles and books available that deal exclusively with this, the medical side of infertility. (RESOLVE and The American Fertility Society always have a good listing of the current writing and research on infertility. See Appendix for addresses.)

THAT FIRST APPOINTMENT

As mentioned before, your specialist will prefer to see both of you. The first reason is to see if both of you feel comfortable with this new medical partner. If so, then he or she will begin by discussing your medical and sexual history individually and as a couple. The doctor will want to know all you've been through. If at all possible, you should bring or have sent any of your medical files pertaining to past infertility work you've done. This usually means you'll have to ask your former doctor in writing for your records. This may sound like a hassle, but it's the best way to get around repeating tests. Besides the fact that it's just no fun to have your blood taken over and over, you'll be paying for all these retakes. Sometimes, however, your doctor will have a good reason to redo a test. You should be open to that.

As for detailed medical history, the doctor will ask questions about your family's health record as well as your own. And he or she will need to know your sexual history: previous pregnancies, information about your menstrual cycle, even questions you may feel to be somewhat intimate in nature. But information about frequency of lovemaking, positions, habits, previous use of contraceptions, lubricants, etc., can help the specialist evaluate what is happening to you as a couple. Sometimes the doctor will even want to interview you separately. You may prefer this. But whatever the situation, be very open and honest. The doctor is on your side. The more correct information doctors have, the better their "detective work" will be.

The doctor will then probably explain the timetable for the work-up. The basic testing can take anywhere from three or four months to a year or more, depending on how fast you want to go. And some treatments may stretch much longer. Because lots of the tests call for perfect timing with your menstrual cycle and perfect patience from the two of you, there will be days you feel that you've created a monster. You *will* have to make the work-up a priority, time-wise. You may have to take off from work, you may have to begin each morning by taking your temperature and end some nights with timed lovemaking. And you may have to juggle all the other areas of your life around those work-up plans. So for mental health's sake, you may want to take it somewhat slower than a textbook might deem worthy. Still, it's up to you and your spouse.

Also realize what you'll be going through. There's no denying that the beginning of an infertility work-up is a powerfully stressful time, for both of you. You'll get a strange feeling you're being tested and scored, that you've passed or failed a "test." A friend of mine put it this way:

I felt like a kid. Did I pass, Doctor? Did I fail? How'd I do? Did we perform all right? Am I adequate? I had the awful feeling every time I saw the doctor that my whole life hinged on the outcome of the latest "exam grade." And that if I didn't produce, I just might be "left behind."

And even stranger, you may begin to wish the doctor would find something wrong with you so he could get on with fixing it.

Following my laparoscopy (a surgical procedure explained later), I can still feel how surreal the whole scene felt as I came out of anaesthesia to hear my doctor whisper, "Good news. . . ."

My first thoughts were, *Good. He's found something wrong. I've got endometriosis or something.*

But his next words were, ". . . There's nothing wrong. You're perfectly normal."

I remember thinking, *That's good news!? That's the same news I've been hearing for years now. And I haven't felt good about it yet!*

It's only natural to feel strange about these tests, and about your reactions to them. Especially since you don't feel sick and yet you're at the hospital or clinic enough to file for permanent residency. It's not unusual for the woman to feel uneasy, embarrassed, angry, even violated, over some of the procedures. And it's not unusual for the man to feel helpless, for most often his tests consist of several minor exams while his wife might have to undergo many costly and somewhat painful procedures. The only protection for such feelings is knowing that they are not wrong or unnatural.

OVERVIEW

Basically, your fertility work-up will be designed around answering four questions. As the American Fertility Society explains it, they are:

- **Is there an egg?** A woman's eggs need to be released regularly.

- **Are there enough sperm?** A man must produce enough active sperm.
- **Can egg and sperm meet?** The egg and sperm must be able to meet.
- **Can implantation occur?** A fertilized egg must implant in the uterus.[22]

As mentioned before, in ninety percent of infertility cases a cause will be found. The most common problems among women are ovulatory problems, scarring or adhesions in the fallopian tubes, and endometriosis (a problem with the uterus lining explained in more detail later).

The most common problems in men are a varicose vein in the scrotum, some sort of testicular failure or ductal obstruction, and problems with sperm count or movement.

PHYSICAL EXAMINATION

It all begins with a good analysis of your basic health. After asking you important questions about long-term medications you may be taking, about your intake of alcohol and drugs, even about your exposure to toxic chemicals, your doctor will begin a physical exam.

A woman should expect a thorough pelvic exam. Much can be told from the size, shape, position, and condition of a woman's pelvic organs. And most doctors will continue to do this exam off and on all through the work-up months. Also, routine blood and urine tests will be taken to check your general health, probably including a Pap smear.

For the man, the exam will consist of the same sort of routine blood and urine tests plus examination of the genital organs, examination of size, position, condition of the penis and testicles. A rectal exam will also be in order. Usually a urologist will do this examination so that he can check for varicose veins, a problem called "varicocele," and other such unsuspected problems. If you are seeing an infertility specialist or a gynecologist, he or she will almost certainly suggest a urologist to consult for this examination. Since the examination on the male is fairly simple, pains should be taken to be sure that nothing is missed, and that a competent doctor is doing the examining.[23]

TESTING FOR THE MAN

Until recently, male infertility was underestimated and undertreated, mainly due to the total lack of expertise or knowledge about it. As George Tagatz, director of the infertility clinic at the University of Minnesota Medical Center, sums it up: "If ever there was an area of medicine in which a great deal of empiricism and witchcraft is practiced, it's male infertility."[22] Except for surgery to repair blockage of sperm delivery, including more and more successful attempts at vasectomy reversals, male infertility treatment still consists mainly of a thorough semen analysis and largely experimental therapies such as taking fertility drugs. Besides that, the man might be advised to deny himself saunas and nylon running shorts (when low sperm count is affected by heat), but, overall, that's about it. Therefore, such a short work-up just makes the semen analysis all the more important.

The first step in any infertility work-up should be this simple test—the semen analysis. Before the wife is put through all the expensive, uncomfortable, even somewhat risky tests, the couple should first find out if the husband is fertile. There are some men who may at first refuse such a test for reasons ranging from feeling strongly negative about what he must do to gain the specimen to worrying about his masculinity if the test shows him sterile. Yet, this analysis is very basic, very important, and *must* be done. Considering what the wife may have to go through, it's a very small thing to ask.

The analysis is, in effect, a "sperm count," but it's much more than that. Not all laboratories are equipped to do a decent job in evaluation of this test. Errors and misinterpretations can easily happen, which is another reason to begin your medical work-up with a specialist or at least a qualified gynecologist and urologist. Much of the analysis' success is based on how the specimen is collected. You'll be told to abstain from love-making for forty-eight to seventy-two hours before the test. Ideally, the husband will collect *all* the sperm specimen into a sterile, large-mouthed jar given to him by the doctor. (If much of it is lost, you may be told to try again later.) No lubricants, such as creams, oil, or soap should be used. And the specimen has to get to the laboratory within one hour of collecting it, making sure it has been kept at body temperature away from heat or cold exposure. Often the doctor will insist that the specimen be collected on the spot so it can be tested immediately. But it can be collected at home if you can make it to the lab within the hour time period.[25]

In one of its articles on the subject, RESOLVE states that since there are people whose religious beliefs prohibit the act of masturbation, other methods can be tried. Your doctor will know about a special nonspermicidal condom that could be used to take a specimen that would be transferred quickly to a jar. And even the post-coital test, explained later, is some-times substituted. None of these alternatives, though, are fool-proof. So considering the important nature of this test, serious thought should be given to coping with this situation by seeing it, first and last, as the medical test it is—if at all possible.

When the lab finally gets the specimen, it will look for the number of sperm present, how fast they are swimming (mo-tility), the shape of the sperm (morphology), the total volume of the specimen, and its thickness (viscosity). A specimen is considered fertile if it has at least twenty million sperm with at least fifty percent of the sperm motile, fifty to sixty percent with good morphology, and a normal volume of 1.5–5 cc. One normal test, though, will not keep you from having to repeat the test, at least one more time, since all the levels fluctuate.[26]

But even if the number, motility, morphology, and viscosity of the semen all check out normal, there still may be a problem. That is why the sperm should also be checked for clumping and agglutination, two possible indicators of "sperm antibody" problems. This is a procedure that calls for special diagnosis capabilities to be read correctly, and many doctors, especially infertility specialists, will take great pains to use labs they can trust.[27]

After my husband's umpteenth semen analysis, I remember overhearing a lab technician somewhat crudely telling my gynecologist that my husband was so fertile he could impregnate a whole harem. This was going on our third year of testing, our post-coital tests weren't looking good, and he was going through the extra semen analysis because an antibody problem had finally been detected. So, again, much weight should be put on how the test is done and interpreted.

TESTING FOR THE WOMAN

BBT—Basal Body Temperature

Your doctor will almost assuredly hand you a chart and tell you to buy a basal body thermometer as he explains how taking your temperature can help predict when you are ovulating. A woman who has a twenty-six to thirty-four-day cycle probably ovulates normally, but you can't be sure. Most doctors believe that the easiest, subjective way to detect whether you ovulate, and maybe when, is to keep a BBT chart. Even though there are some more accurate new at-home methods already being used using urine testing (discussed later), the BBT charting is still the cheapest and easiest, and your doctor will probably want you to include it in your work-up.

Every morning, before you move a muscle, before you turn over, before you turn off the alarm, before *anything*, you—the wife—will take your temperature and record it on the chart. The night before, you have checked your thermometer and laid it close to your bed. Supposedly, the day or two before or after ovulation there is a dip of .2–.5 degrees in a woman's temperature. This is usually above 98 F. (But in my personal case, my temperature was never higher than 97 F. the whole time I used the BBT, and my dip put me into the 96.5 F. range. So take into account your specific situation.) In a few days, due to progesterone, body temperature will rise, not to drop again until the woman's period begins—or if the woman's pregnant, not at all. You and your doctor may attempt to use this to help you time lovemaking so it will happen as close as possible to your ovulation.[28]

But a lot can affect the temperature. Illness can throw it totally off. Even late hours can affect it. And certainly jumping up in the morning before you remember to take your temperature will wreak havoc with accuracy.

Obviously, then, there is certainly nothing exact about the BBT. And after a few months of charting your temperature, you may want to throw the thermometer across the room in defiance of its daily tyranny. And with the way you'll have to account for your lovemaking by putting little X's in the appropriate boxes on the chart, you'll certainly begin to feel like you're keeping score—and once more wonder if you're measuring up. One friend came to that realization in a strange way:

> As I sat at the kitchen table filling out my BBT chart, getting ready for my monthly doctor's visit, I realized that we hadn't made love but twice that month, both times during *the* week. I suddenly worried about what the doctor would think, what he expected, and what he would say. I poised my pencil over a random box, ready to add a few X's for looks, when a childhood memory flashed through my head. This was *exactly* how I felt before my piano lesson after my usual week of little or no practice. To keep from a certain tongue-lashing and a possible knuckle-rapping, I would *cheat* on my practice sheet. . . . And that was same thing I was feeling pressure to do now! Cheat on my chart! Has it really come to this?!

Even after you tear up the charts, you still may do something called "mental charting." You'll be so knowledgeable about your monthly cycle, so in the habit of thinking about your month in chart form, you'll still be keeping tabs on the "right" days of the month.

Still, before that little thermometer takes over your life, you should see it for what it is: a not-entirely-exact yet helpful tool. I know in my own case I spent years thinking I was ovulating on the first part of *the* week according to my BBT. But I found out only recently I seem to ovulate at the end, three to four days later.

As Dr. Stephen Corson explains in his book, *Conquering Infertility:*

> The value of the BBT lies more in its ability to document that ovulation has taken place than in predicting when it will occur. It has long been assumed that ovulation occurs when the BBT chart shows its lowest temperature reading. But recent laboratory tests have shown that ovulation may actually occur two or three days after the lowest reading.[29]

Ideally, then the BBT should be looked on as a diagnostic tool, not a chart to live or die by.

Tests for Ovulation

Other ways to test ovulation are an *endometrial biopsy* in which a tissue sample is surgically removed from the uterine lining for examination (an office procedure that calls for mild sedation); a *serum progesterone* blood test; and a series of *ultra-sounds*, non-surgical examinations using a machine that turns reflected sound waves—that can detect maturing eggs—into pictures on a TV screen.[30] Also, the newest ovulation test, an *LH (hormone) surge urine test*, is a home "dipstick" exam that helps pinpoint ovulation through examining urine for ovulation's hormone surges.[31] Such home exams help you monitor your "LH surge," somewhat like a litmus test. Ovulation usually occurs twenty-four to thirty-six hours following that first LH surge. Your specialist may suggest you use one of these to help pinpoint your ovulation as close as possible and will probably give you a professional kit to use. Also, simpler test kits that are not quite as exact are now being sold over the counter.

Clomiphene Citrate—Clomid

Often, if your doctor suspects that the woman's irregular periods are getting in the way of conception, he or she will prescribe *Clomiphene Citrate (Clomid)* therapy to go with the BBT. Clomid is a truly mild fertility pill that essentially stimulates your ovaries to work like clock-work. It's usually taken on days five through nine of your cycle, and usually given for a minimum of six months, assuming that ovulation was accomplished. And some therapies that include its use may go on much longer. You'll probably start off with a low dose, because women respond differently to Clomid, and there may be certain side effects. That possibility is why your doctor will have you come in monthly for Clomid "checks" while you are using this medication.

Clomid is seen overall as another safe "tool" for battling infertility. As for it being a "fertility pill," only in a low percentage of cases does using it result in multiple births.[32]

H.M.G.—Pergonal

H.M.G., which stands for human menopausal gonadotropin, (*Pergonal*) is the powerful fertility drug made from a natural hormone that's been used since the '60s to force ovulation. (And since 1981, it's been attempted in some male infertility therapy, too.) Its main claims to fame have been its high success rate and its high risk of multiple births. Meticulous monitoring and very careful screening are still the key to successful use of this drug, one reason why only an infertility specialist should undergo the therapy with you. The specialist will probably explore all other possible causes for infertility before starting this therapy, especially checking the prolactin hormone to make sure there is no possibility of the lack of ovulation being caused by a small pituitary tumor.[33]

Pergonal's success rate for producing ovulation is very high, but it's very expensive and it *is* a treatment that requires continual, even daily, observation. As for multiple births, the percentages vary quite a bit, but one study shows that the possibility of having more than one child can be as high as forty-one percent, the majority (seventy-five percent) of those being twins.[34]

Hormonal Testing

These are essentially blood tests. The two hormones that affect ovulation, *FSH* and *LH*, will probably be checked. Both are produced by the pituitary: one, FSH, stimulates the ripening of the egg; the other, LH, stimulates its release. *Thyroid* and *prolactin* levels should be tested. Testosterone and androgen hormones might also be tested if you have very irregular cycles and unusual facial or body hair growth. A test for diabetes might not be out of order, since subtle cases can go undetected and can affect fertility.[35]

Hysterosalpingogram

—A very long word that refers to an X-ray examination of the uterus and fallopian tubes that a radiologist will administer. A special dye that becomes visible on X-ray film is injected into the uterus through the cervix. If everything is normal, the dye will fill the uterus and spill out of the fallopian tubes. If not, this test can spot defects in the uterus or blockage in the tubes. This is a very important but quite uncomfortable test, one that you'll probably need sedation for. And it should only be done in the first part of the menstrual cycle.

One expert warns that a few women might be allergic to the dye since it contains iodine. If you are allergic to shellfish (which contain iodine) you should mention it to your doctor. Also, while most radiologists use a water-based dye, some still use an oil-type dye that could become clogged in blocked tubes. And, as with all X-rays, you should definitely be given only the minimum amount. Occasionally, a patient will develop a pelvic infection after the test—pain, fever, vaginal discharge within a five-day period. If you do, your doctor should be told.

The *hysterosalpingogram* takes the place of the Rubin Test that uses gas pressure.[36]

Post-Coital Test

Your doctor will want to find out how well the husband's sperm survive once they come into contact with his wife's cervical mucus. Your doctor can find out through the *post-coital (Sims-Huhner) test,* which evaluates both cervical mucus (whether enough estrogen is present) and sperm (whether enough "motile" or moving sperm are present). The mucus can be "hostile" in the sense that it prevents sperm from entering the uterus, possibly carrying antibodies that actually kill the sperm on contact. (There is even a cervical mucus antibody test, which many infertility specialists use.)

As for the procedure and timing of the test, it's exactly as it sounds. You will be asked to make love in the morning, or whenever the wife can come directly, within two to three hours, to the doctor's office. There the doctor will take a sample of mucus and study it under a microscope. The test must also be timed to coincide with ovulation so that the quality of the cervical mucus will allow the sperm to move around freely. This may not sound very complicated, but while some women have "good" mucus for days, others have it only for hours.[37]

Again, timing becomes all-important, and a BBT chart can help. To make matters even more complicated, though, opinions differ on exactly how to evaluate the test. I know one couple whose post-coitals were continually poor over a matter of years. It was really the only test they could show that wasn't normal through their whole work-up. Yet, suddenly one month they turned up pregnant.

Our poor result in this test, though, was one of the factors that pointed us toward reevaluating that old sperm antibody test, which led us to find our antibody problem.

Laparoscopy

This is a surgical procedure, usually done on an outpatient, same-day level, but most of the time using general anaesthesia and all that goes with that. In other words, it shouldn't be taken lightly. Yet, the *laparoscopy* is the latest in the quite amazing new diagnostic work connected to infertility. It's all but replaced tests similar in nature but not as effective or as easy, such as the culdoscopy. Laparoscopy is a procedure in which a tiny, lighted telescope is inserted through the navel to allow the doctor to actually view the outside of the uterus, the tubes, and the ovaries. It is integral in checking the presence of scar tissue around the tubes or ovaries, and also for detecting endometriosis.[38]

Endometriosis is quite a common condition in which the endometrial tissue that lines the uterus begins to connect and grow in all the wrong places. It's become a modern day, albeit mysterious, problem, the only symptoms being painful periods and infertility. But even that's not always the case. There may be no symptoms at all. Ultimately, the only way to know for sure is to undergo the laparoscopy.

If there is endometriosis, all is not lost. More and more cases can be treated and more and more pregnancies are made possible. Doctors treat it with a drug called danazol, a synthetic male hormone that stops ovulation and causes endometrial tissue to shrivel. Experimental treatments are also now being done with a substance called nafarelin.

For severe cases of endometriosis, surgery may be suggested. A procedure called videolaseroscopy, which employs a laparoscope rigged with a tiny video camera and a laser, is a high-tech type of surgery that has been quite successful in recent applications.[39]

SPERM ANTIBODIES

After all these tests, you might possibly still come up "normal," or, in other words, none of the tests will have detected any problem. The next step is to suspect some sort of *immunological* problem—you might be producing *antibodies*, in your blood or in your mucus, against your spouse or even against yourself.

Even though this problem sounds a little weird, believe it or not, "haywire" antibody reactions are quite common. An ordinary case of hay fever or allergy is a good example. Transplant patients must cope with this wrong-thinking, built-in defense mechanism.

Actually, when you think about it, a woman *should* form antibodies against sperm, since they are after all quite foreign to her body. But only a very small percentage of infertile women have this "allergic" reaction to sperm. Those who do may form antibodies against all sperm, or strangely enough, only against their mates' sperm. As for men, the situation is about the same. Men who have had vasectomies sometimes are found to produce antibodies against their own sperm. But some men who've never had a vasectomy will still produce antibodies against their own sperm.[40]

The reason's aren't clear, and the testing isn't much clearer. The sperm antibody test is a blood test that can show whether you as a couple are producing antibodies against one another, or you as individuals are producing them against yourselves. The antibody test can also be done on cervical mucus. Antibodies may show up in the mucus or in the sperm but not in the blood. Poor post-coital tests, as mentioned above, will suggest this problem—although they aren't terribly reliable—as will the agglutination test done during the semen analysis.

Yet all through this, the man's sperm count can be perfectly normal. Very few labs are doing all the immunological diagnoses. And different specialists trust different labs, which not only adds to the confusion but underscores the uneasy feeling about this whole problem.

The treatments aren't much more clear. One treatment for a woman's antibody problem is actually to use birth control! It's called "condom therapy" and the idea is to give the woman time for the level of antibodies to lower before attempting conception again.[41] Another treatment, for the man, is to use steroids to suppress the immune system thereby suppressing the antibodies. But the inherent risks may not be worth the effort. In high doses, they can cause ulcers, diabetes, and other undesirable things. And if the man is on any sort of medication, high blood pressure medicine for instance, taking steroids may even be more undersirable.

But even though modern medicine is coming up with ways to attempt combat with the immune system when it gets in the way of fertility, the question marks are still large on what relationship the immune system and infertility have with one another.

SPERM WASHING AND A.I.H.

Two other methods are being used more and more for antibody problems. *A.I.H.-artificial insemination with husband's sperm* (also called intrauterine insemination) is a procedure that is also being tried for situations such as low sperm count, poor motility, poor cervical mucus, poor post-coital tests, and even cases of unexplained infertility.

For antibody problems, A.I.H. is coupled with *sperm washing*, or sperm processing, a technique in which the sperm cells are separated from the seminal fluid by gentle centrifugal force. The process is repeated over and over, sperm counts being taken at each step. Finally the sperm are suspended in a small volume of embryo medium, the same liquid used to grow embryos during in vitro (test tube) fertilization. The process takes several hours, then is coupled with A.I.H. during which the husband's washed sperm will be placed inside the uterus or cervix by the specialist.

Of course, like all the other tests, timing is all-important—maybe more so in this case, because the whole process is useless if it doesn't coincide perfectly with the wife's ovulation. Ultrasounds may be prescribed during the two or three times during the month you will attempt the A.I.H. sperm washing in an attempt to match the washings with the ovulation as close as humanly possible. Since it can actually see the egg mature inside its "follicle," the ultrasound can help predict by the follicle's size when it will be ready.[42] The LH surge urine test described earlier can also help in the timing, in tandem with ultrasounds, or often in lieu of them, because the inseminations could be scheduled about twenty-four hours after the surge.

If you've gone this far in the work-up, you'll probably shake your head in disbelief at how complicated the whole experience has become. If you are having the A.I.H./sperm washing procedure done, your pinpointed week during the month will probably start at daybreak when you'll obtain the specimen, rush it to the lab, then twiddle your thumbs for an average of three to five hours it takes to wash the sperm.

A.I.H./sperm washing, though, is often a logical and somewhat therapeutic resort. Odds of pregnancy are about the same as the average couple on the average month—about twenty percent.[43] But if you are among the couples who have had no odds at all, that twenty percent looks pretty good. Specialists have a growing list of situations that A.I.H./sperm washings might help, and they will want to try the procedure with you for several months before calling it quits.

Then, if none of these basic procedures help you toward that elusive thing called conception, modern medicine has some modern alternatives.

BASIC WORK-UP CHECKLIST

MALE TESTING

_____ Physical

_____ Semen analysis

FEMALE TESTING/TREATMENT

_____ Physical

_____ Testing for Ovulation

    _____ BBT charts

    _____ cervical check

    _____ Serum progesterone

    _____ Endometrial biopsy

    _____ LH surge urine test

    _____ Ultrasound

_____ Clomiphene Citrate (Clomid) therapy

_____ Hormone testing

    _____ thyroid

    _____ prolactin

    _____ FSH/LH

    _____ estrogen/progesterone

    _____ testosterone/androgen

_____ Hysterosalpingogram

_____ Laparoscopy

_____ Pergonal therapy

COMBINED TESTING/TREATMENT

_____ Post-coital (Sims-Huhner) tests

_____ Immunological testing

    _____ blood test—sperm antibody

    _____ mucus test—sperm antibody

_____ Sperm washing and A.I.H.

THE MEDICAL WORK-UP—THE COMPLEX PROCEDURES

BRAVE NEW WORLD TODAY

They make headlines everyday somewhere in the world—test tube fertilization, embryo transfer, sperm banks, artificial insemination, surrogate mothers—the amazing, unnerving new methods that have been conjured up through mixing biology and technology.

And amazing is truly the word for what has happened during the last ten years. This biotechnological explosion has ushered us into a new era. Besides the sensational procedures that are dotting the media and causing legal and ethical headaches, though, medicine has also been steadily at work producing other creative approaches to infertility:

- microsurgery using miniaturized tools to open blocked or scarred tubes and sperm ducts, even reverse vasectomies
- laser surgery for endometriosis
- hormone therapies that induce ovulation
- sonogram testing—using sound waves, ultrasound, for monitoring of the egg development on the ovaries

Add those to the new headline-grabbing alternatives and we can't help but feel we are living in the future. Every day seems to show us some new medical advance followed by some new social complication. It's a crazy world we live in, full of the beautiful and the horrifying. And sometimes the two get mixed up.

As science keeps unraveling the secret of nature's reproduction process—which is in essence what it is doing—we'll see more and more of the amazing. So, no matter what your personal point of view, you as a couple facing infertility will be touched by all of this brave new world paraphernalia. And you need to have at least a light grasp of what these procedures are. That way, if you do find yourselves presented with these options down the infertility road, you can bring a decent amount of knowledge to your decision of what is right or wrong for you medically, and then morally. First, let's explain what these new procedures are.

MICRO SURGERY AND LASER SURGERY

Both of these new procedures are slowly and surely taking the place of "macrosurgery," normal surgical procedures. With all the new miniaturization of instruments going on, *microsurgery* is truly a wave of the future that is happening now. Its use of miniaturized microscopes and tools can help overcome the damage that infections wreak on fallopian tubes and the pelvis area—easier, quicker, cleaner.

Laser surgery as in the "videolaseroscopy" mentioned earlier, is actually a lot like you'd picture it. The laser's beam "zaps" the endometrial growth out of existence, leaving very little bleeding. This is the same sort of technology that has revolutionized eye surgery in recent years.

THE FERTILITY PUMP

When a woman's infertility stems from her brain not giving off the right signals for production of the pituitary-stimulating hormone, doctors can actually attach an experimental *fertility pump* to her that injects a synthetic form of the hormone all through the day. So far, experimental statistics show a high success of ovulation, and even a few pregnancies.[44]

A.I.D.—ARTIFICIAL INSEMINATION BY DONOR

A.I.D. is different from A.I.H., discussed earlier, in one very big way. The sperm is from a donor instead of the husband.

When all else fails in the treatment of male infertility, then A.I.D. becomes an alternative. And even though it has its controversial overtones, estimates suggest that just in America there are over ten thousand babies conceived this way each year. And the number could be drastically more. S. J. Behrman, a nationally acclaimed infertility specialist, estimates the figure at closer to fifty thousand births a year. But because no separate birth records are kept on A.I.D. children, any estimate is just an educated guess.[45] Either number, though, inspires incredulity. How could a procedure be so widely used yet keep such a low profile? And even more surprising is the fact that it's a procedure that's been used commonly for thirty years, and dates back to the end of the nineteenth century.

Why would a couple consider such a drastic move? This is a valid question, especially since, obviously, so many do. Several answers probably could be given to that question. Each year, more than a million American men are sterilized by vasectomy. But more men than you imagine decide they want children after the fact, for many reasons. In this age of divorce, a man who's had a vasectomy may be going into a second marriage and may want to begin a new family. The same situation might happen if his first wife dies and he remarries. Or maybe he realizes, too late, that his vasectomy was a wrong decision. For a grab bag of reasons, he might put himself through vasectomy reversal surgery. For those men whose reversals are unsuccessful, they and their wives may seriously consider A.I.D. as an option. Also, the cost of the expensive operation might make the reversal financially impossible, so A.I.D. becomes even more a possible alternative.

Some couples who know that the husband carries a dominant or recessive trait for an inheritable disease such as hemophilia or cystic fibrosis might choose A.I.D. over natural conception rather than risk passing on the disease.

But most of all, consider the couple who has antibody problems or whose husband is sterile, or even those who've gone for years without any reason at all for the infertility. If they decide to continue pursuing their quest for a baby, they might apply for adoption only to find that it will be a two to five year wait—or worse, to find that they are continually turned down because of age or other medical problems. Infertility provides enough feelings of failure and blows to self-esteem. To be told you aren't quality material for adoption is unbelievably cruel. But it happens. And it will happen even more as the number of available unwanted babies decreases, inevitably making the adoption standards more and more selective. What does such a couple do? Our culture puts a high premium on parenting and procreation. There is pressure from within and from without to have a child, to be a parent, to have a family. So many couples, as the adoption situation becomes tighter, will look elsewhere, like to A.I.D., for fulfillment of that desire.

One of the most frustrating side effects of modern living affecting the infertile couple is today's adoption situation. Abortion, wide-spread birth control use, and our society's openness to unmarried mothers have made adoption a game of desperate wait-and-hope-and-see, instead of a gesture of sensitive humanity. In times past, adoption might have been especially attractive to those infertile couples who felt they might be giving an unwanted child a home and love. But with today's severe shortage of available babies, the focus is no longer on the unwanted child, but on the unneeded parent.

So, again, for the couple who's just been through years of infertility stress, the adoption process can be just another form of the same elusive search, another cruel quirk of modern life. Such couples might begin to view A.I.D. as a form of adoption, a sort of "adopt a sperm." Since conventional adoption has become so selective, some people see their only choice being, in a sense, to adopt the baby at a much earlier stage—prior to conception. In doing so they can control at least half the situation—the child would be biologically closer to the parents, emotionally and physically. And the couple can also experience pregnancy and childbirth together, even nursing, if the woman wants.[46]

Such couples might see other advantages of A.I.D. over adoption. The complicated legal machinery involving social workers, lawyers, and doctors—many of whom continue hovering over the adoptive family for quite awhile—would not exist. And that elusive fear many adoptive parents have that the baby's natural mother might at any moment show up to claim the baby would not be a factor either. Usually the man's infertility is only known by the couple and their doctor, and the anonymity of the donor is highly guarded.

Reasons vary for contemplating A.I.D. and they are almost always deeply personal. But most clinics will make counseling mandatory, often with an on-staff social worker or psychiatrist, before allowing a couple into an A.I.D. program. The man's self-image must be healthy for him to grapple with the idea that the child is not biologically his; the woman might feel in some way that she is not being faithful, especially since she pays for the effort; both must decide if they will tell anyone including the possible child. And the couple must decide how desperately essential they believe a child is to their marital happiness, because there's no turning back. It is definitely not a procedure that the man should undergo for the sake of his wife. Any hesitancy at all should be reason enough not to try this alternative, or to at least wait or seek counseling on such a life-shaping decision.

Medically, A.I.D. is a fairly successful and more common procedure than you might imagine. The same sort of emphasis on timing and on ovulation needed in A.I.H. is needed in A.I.D. If the woman hasn't gone through the basic infertility tests, she may be told she must go through some of them in order to time her ovulation, to make sure she has no inheritable diseases herself, besides checking to see if she has any other problems. Since such work-ups entail a month or two, the couple will also have a while to reevaluate their decision. The specialist will probably want to try the procedure at least six times or so before abandoning the effort.[47]

But the major questions about A.I.D. involve the donor.

Who is this person? Why would he want to do such a thing? How is he picked? The awesome responsibility of picking a donor rests on the shoulders of the specialist and his staff. The larger the program the better, since the pool of qualified donors must necessarily be near and willing to be called at any time. In many programs, pains will be taken to match blood type, skin, height, physical features, and, at some special sperm banks, even interests and aptitudes. The donor is screened— his sperm, his background, his medical and family histories, his present health through blood tests. (Often, medical students are donors because of their close proximity and probable mental, intellectual, and physical stability.) But, whoever they are, they are always anonymous, and usually stay that way. Each program has its own restrictions, but most take great care to keep records in a place where even medical staff members cannot find them. They may also destroy them after a set amount of time. Anonymity, then, is the highest priority for most A.I.D. programs.

As for why a man would want to donate his sperm, money is the obvious answer, even though many of those asked express a very real sense of helping, giving the gift of a baby to couples who might never have one otherwise. This point remains one of the grayer areas of this alternative, especially when few restrictions are placed on the times a donor is used and the quality of records kept.

And when the courts become involved with a medical procedure, you know it's no simple one. Most states now make the husband and wife both sign a consent form that makes the husband the legal guardian of the child. And that's only one of the legal aspects being studied and acted upon in the use of A.I.D. With the possible ethical questions involved, A.I.D. becomes even more complicated. Morally, philosophically, and religiously, A.I.D. is difficult for many couples to accept. (Many of A.I.D.'s legal, social, and ethical dimensions will be discussed in Section 4.)

Artificial insemination by donor is still a controversial issue, even though legally the problems are being addressed and ethically they are now being pondered. Much more needs to be considered past the actual procedure. Contemplating A.I.D. truly calls for a time of self-evaluation, of marital evaluation, of value clarification, of serious study. Then, if you decide to undergo A.I.D., great care should obviously be taken in picking a program, one linked to a teaching hospital or to a reputable infertility clinic so that there can be no question about the quality of the program. (Again, RESOLVE and the American Fertility Society, as mentioned earlier, are good sources of information about reputable A.I.D. programs. See Appendix.)

SPERM BANKS/EMBRYO BANKS/EGG BANKS

"Life is in a sense a series of chemical events proceeding irreversibly toward death, and these chemical events cannot take place at -400°," states Sherman Silber, as he explains sperm freezing and sperm banks (or "cryobanks").[48] In veterinary work today, sperm freezing is common, used continually in breeding. For humans, the first reason for using frozen sperm for infertility problems was the idea that by freezing sperm, a husband with a low sperm count could keep adding to a frozen sperm bank "account," until he had enough to artificially inseminate his wife. But it doesn't work. Research has found that so far only a minority of all men have sperm that can survive being frozen. And sperm from infertile men do even more poorly, dying quickly in such a frozen state.[49]

But as for healthy sperm, babies have been born through A.I.D. using sperm that have been frozen. Most infertility clinics and teaching hospitals don't have the complex facilities it takes to have a sperm bank. But some major ones do, and the A.I.D. practitioners see such a "saving" procedure as a convenient one. The woman can be inseminated whenever her cycle dictates without worrying about having the donor on call.

The same idea, having supply on hand, can be applied to freezing eggs as well as freezing embryos—and *has* been, with success, by the precedent-setting in vitro fertilization program at Queen Victoria Hospital in Melbourne, Australia.[50] Most in vitro fertilization ("test tube fertilization") specialists would like the use of frozen embryos or eggs to avoid surgery on the woman every time she must go through the procedure. (These new procedures, however, are already having their own strange ethical twists, such as the one in which two frozen embryos were suddenly "orphaned" when the woman from whom the eggs were taken was killed in a plane crash along with her husband. A committee had to be set up to decide what to do with the frozen embryos.)[51]

IN VITRO FERTILIZATION

In 1978, an Englishwoman named Leslie Brown decided to try a last ditch effort. She and her husband had been married nine years and couldn't have children because her tubes were so badly destroyed by scars and inflammation that even microsurgery couldn't help her. Her ovaries and uterus were okay, though, so all that was really required to grant her wish for a baby was to take an egg from one of her ovaries, combine it with her husband's sperm in a dish until it became fertilized, and then implant the fertilized egg—the embryo—back into her womb where it could grow into a full-term baby. There was just one catch. It had never been successfully done before.

But the Browns took the chance anyway, and on July 25, 1978 their daughter Louise Brown was born—and one of the most sensational controversies of the century began dotting our newspapers and news shows. Some called it a great scientific breakthrough, others insisted it was an irreverent interference with nature, and the controversy rages on. Drs. Robert Edwards and Patrick Steptoe had spent twelve years of research toward that one day, and we have no idea where it will lead us. But the one thing any infertile couple will hear above all the din is hope—there is now an alternative to some otherwise hopeless cases.[52]

In 1981, the first American baby was born through in vitro (also called I.V.F.). Popularly called "test-tube fertilization," the procedure actually takes place in a shallow dish, "in vitro" literally meaning "in glass" in Latin. Instead of happening inside a woman's body, the conception—when the sperm and the egg meet—happens outside the body.[53]

And so the actual reference to Aldous Huxley's 1946 futuristic classic *Brave New World*, in which babies literally grow full term in test tubes, is slightly off, but still colorful. However, there's no denying that the reference, in its heralding of the impossible becoming probable, is symbolically on target.

Explained briefly, in vitro happens this way: After meticulous timing and probable Clomid or Pergonal therapy, the woman usually undergoes a laparoscopy in which the doctor takes eggs from her ovary and places them in a special culture medium in a glass dish. The husband will at the same time provide semen, which probably will go through sperm washing before being added to the eggs in the culture dish. If all goes well, the sperm will fertilize the egg (or eggs). The doctors will watch the embryos for about forty hours, then will examine the egg. If everything looks normal, the fertilized egg will be transferred into the woman's uterus about forty-eight hours after the laparoscopy. Then it's hoped that the embryo will adhere to the lining of the uterus and grow until a healthy baby is born.[54] And we'll read about it in the morning edition. But since the number of babies born compared to the number of attempts is *extremely* low, we know that all does not always go well.

Well, then, what about success rates? How often do things *not* go well? The fertilization success rates, of the eggs and sperm in the glass dish, are reported to be high. But after that, it's downhill. The success of the transfer and the implantation into the uterus of the new embryo has been very, very low. For most clinics, the rate is about twenty percent at best, ten to fifteen percent more realistically. And for the last step, carrying the baby fullterm, the success rate is not much higher. The more successful clinics experience around twenty to thirty percent at best, (about the same as the natural rate).[55] And as more and more new clinics pop up around the country, the individual clinic rate will probably become even lower. Some clinics may wait through thirty to forty or more attempts before achieving a pregnancy—and even more for a baby.[56] The American Fertility Society reports that more than half of the country's clinics have yet to experience a single birth.[57]

Opinions vary on success rates, because "success' is defined in different ways by different clinics. For some clinics, it's pregnancy, even if miscarriage is the end result. For others, it is the birth of a live baby. And another aspect of the success issue is that it may also vary with the number of embryos transferred. The success rate goes up with the number of embryos—in other words, if one embryo has about ten percent chance of successfully implanting into the uterus, two embryos make for a twenty percent, and on up it goes. So to boost the possible success rate, a clinic, more than not, will opt to induce superovulation to obtain more embryos to transfer.[58]

In other words, there is a lot we are not told about I.V.F. As you investigate I.V.F. possibilities and as I.V.F. techniques are improved, you may hear higher success rate percentages, but be careful to ask what the success rate is based upon. Some clinics even add what they call "chemical pregnancies" that only last a few days to their success rate quote. In this way, these clinics can brag of, say, a twenty percent success rate when they have never even had a live birth! And yet that's the only "success" we want to know about—a live birth.[59] One of the most successful American clinics boasts that thirty-eight percent of all women who come to see them become pregnant.[60] All of these pregnancies may go fullterm, but it's doubtful, and anyone considering I.V.F. should ask for a clinic's "live birth" percentage—how many of the women who become pregnant actually walk out of the clinic with that "miracle" baby.

So, question marks dot the "success" rates, and the ways they're interpreted. And yet hopes are raised by such rates—the infertile couple will hear only the higher rate no matter how it is defined. And that in itself can be cruel. Researchers, of course, are continually working to improve the odds. As for now, though, I.V.F. is still, as one science writer called it, a "costly long shot." Anyone contemplating I.V.F. must take all this into consideration.

Who, specifically, can I.V.F. help? Because of the research nature of the procedure, you don't just walk into an infertility clinic and ask for an appointment. In fact, you must apply and wait. And though there may be many teaching hospitals and clinics trying the procedure, success rates vary from hospital to hospital, and clinic to clinic some still waiting for their first success story. As one specialist put it, in vitro clinics are only as good as their Ph.D. in biology who works with the glass dish fertilization step.

Obviously, I.V.F. cannot be for everyone. Many clinics have age limits, some only accepting women who are infertile due to totally blocked or destroyed fallopian tubes. Lately, many clinics have also been accepting women with endometriosis, a history of ectopic (out of the uterus) pregnancies, cervical mucus problems, and even "normal"—unexplained—infertility. However, all of the clinics require that the women have one workable, accessible ovary, which usually means that the woman must undergo a laparoscopy just to qualify. To stave off any possibility of birth defects, most women will be required to show some form of immunity to German measles, which if caught during pregnancy can cause such defects. And the man, of course, must show a healthy semen analysis.

Very little, though, is said about the rigors of going through the process, which includes many days away from home and work at a time and at a moment's notice, an involved medical ordeal, days in bed following each attempt, and on and on.[61] (To get a realistic picture of the rigors involved with I.V.F., read such personal experience articles as the one quoted in endnote 56.)

But the worst hurdle is probably the most unfair one— money. The cost of the procedure itself is exorbitant—latest figures showing from three to eight thousand dollars. And since there is no restriction on the number of times a couple can try I.V.F., some have tried five times or more, even though the success rate does not increase with more times tried. A little figuring on your calculator will tell you that the costs of the procedure can accumulate into a small fortune. And because of infertility's experimental and "nonlife-threatening" status, most insurance presently will not cover any of the procedure.

(Recently, Massachusetts Blue Cross/Blue Shield decided to cover it and Maryland law requires its state's insurance companies to cover I.V.F.[62] So things are looking up.) Furthermore, most I.V.F. clinics will require that the entire amount be paid in advance. Add the cost of traveling, hotel rooms, time off from work—time that could run into a week or more for each attempt—and that figure becomes untouchable for the average couple.[63]

The overriding emotions connected to the procedure, once again, cannot be overemphasized. The chances are low. The cost is high. If the procedure doesn't work anywhere along the chain of events, the couple is usually made to wait several months before trying again. And just waiting your turn may have lasting emotional dangers. For example, at the Norfolk, Virginia clinic, there has been a backlog of about one-thousand women wanting I.V.F. A sad by-product of such a wait is expressed by Martin Quigley, now with the Cleveland Clinic Foundation. Commenting on his work with the University of Texas Health Sciences Center's I.V.F. program, he said: "By the time our program was operational, two years after we started taking applications, half of the first couples on our waiting list had separated or divorced."[64]

Although I.V.F. may become commonplace in the future, currently it's loaded down with many considerations past the medical miracle it is. The reason, for instance, that the Department of Health, Education, and Welfare placed a moratorium on federal funds for I.V.F. research was due to ethical questions about the whole area of technology. High cost, low success rates, long waiting lines, ethical questions—such considerations continue to make I.V.F. a procedure of last resort. It is an amazing new development in infertility research, but the couple thinking about pursuing it should go into it with their eyes wide open. As the Oregon Health Sciences University explains in their pamphlet on their own I.V.F. program:

> Couples who are considering I.V.F. should realize that it is an intensely emotional, physically arduous, and expensive procedure

with a small chance of success. Most couples find it difficult to look at the chances for success realistically without dampening the drive that allows them to undertake I.V.F. Above all, couples should explore plans for the future, regardless of whether or not their attempt at I.V.F. is successful.[65]

OTHER POTENTIAL TECHNIQUES THROUGH THE NEW BIOTECHNOLOGY

All of these new procedures open doors to even further sensational, and maybe questionable, possibilities:

What if a couple has had trouble coaxing sperm and egg to meet in the body's natural incubator, the fallopian tubes? Maybe there have been cervical problems, or low sperm count or poor sperm motility—even, again, "normal" infertility. Usually they would be prime candidates for I.V.F., but other ideas are popping up. A promising potential alternative that might bypass some of I.V.F.'s inherent problems is "Gamet intra-fallopian transfer," or G.I.F.T. G.I.F.T. is a procedure in which the sperm and eggs are placed in the fallopian tubes, instead of in a dish, to fertilize. Supposedly, the chief advantage of the procedure is that it relies more on the body's natural process to produce pregnancy. And of course, it would not require the time and should not require the exorbitant costs of I.V.F. In contrast to I.V.F., it would be an alternative only for women with healthy fallopian tubes.[66] As G.I.F.T. begins to produce better and better success rates, rivaling and bettering I.V.F.'s., more and more hospitals will be looking at its worth.

What if a woman can't produce an egg, but otherwise could carry a baby to term? One answer could be *embryo transfer*, the opposite of A.I.D. Instead of donor sperm, there is a donor egg. An egg would be extracted from a donor through a laparoscopy, fertilized with her husband's sperm through I.V.F., and placed in her uterus.

What if a women has had a hysterectomy, but still has normal ovaries and a fertile husband? It's now possible to remove one of her eggs through laparoscopy, fertilize it in vitro, then implant it into another woman: a *surrogate mother.*

Possibly one of the most explosive issues in this infertility debate has to be this idea of surrogate motherhood. Legally and ethically, it is very controversial, to say the least. Basically, surrogating is a contractual relationship between a couple who want a child but who cannot have one because of the woman's infertility and a woman willing to bear the husband's child for them. (That's surrogating in its simplest form. As we will discuss in the next section, "hi-tech" surrogating is already happening, one example being that the surrogate "mother" is only an incubator of sorts for an embryo fertilized in vitro with a couple's egg and sperm.) Actual programs are in existence which bring these two factions together, sometime taking care of everything from the insemination, to prenatal care, to delivery costs, to legal costs.[67] The problems are obvious and many. Its legality is definitely under question. (A British ethics board commissioned by Parliament has recommended making such private agencies dealing in surrogating absolutely illegal.)[68]

At the present time, these programs are neither legal or illegal, which puts the whole idea in limbo. The high price tag on surrogating, twenty-five thousand dollars and up, makes it an alternative only for the very rich. Yet even after all is paid and done, present contracts cannot in actuality be seen as legally binding. So anything can happen.[69]

And this is one of the many areas where ethics as well as law comes into play. What does the couple do if the woman decides not to give up the newborn? What if the baby is deformed? What if the couple decides they don't want the baby? Such cases are already happening, and we'll discuss them in more detail in the next section.

Legal or not, and ethical or not, surrogating is already happening today. But it is not a procedure that will, anytime soon, overcome its all-around inherently questionable aspects.

And questionable may also be the term for the other techniques involved with the today's biotechnological explosion.

Add *genetic selection*, *sex selection*, and *embryo banks* to our choices, and believe it or not, ready or not, these options are unfolding now. Even transplants—ovaries, fallopian tubes, testes—are not unthinkable.

Today's biotechnology affords us, or will afford us, all these alternatives and more to choose from—and all their inherent issues to ponder. Most infertile couples will welcome any help, no matter how complicated or expensive or even questionable, with open arms. Again, the question may become "What price a baby?" as science begins to carry us along that thin line between ethics and medicine.

"If this treatment doesn't work," the specialist is saying, "there are still alternatives. Have you thought about them at all?"

Wearily, I lean back against the examining table. "Alternatives," I repeat. "You mean like artificial insemination by a donor, or test tube fertilization or something?

"Well, yes."

I already knew that this hospital had a donor program, and I already knew that my former specialist had left to work with an in vitro fertilization clinic. I knew all that. But not until this moment had "all that" ever been offered as something personal. Something desperately, intimately, agonizingly personal . . .

"We'll see. We've still got a decent chance with this treatment," he is saying as he jots down today's notes. "Oh, I did hear that an in vitro specialist is speaking tonight in your town. Had you heard?"

"Yes. I heard something about it."

"You might want to go hear him. He is highly respected. It's a fascinating field. And it never hurts to be informed." He looks up and smiles. "But as for us, let's not worry about other procedures quite yet. You are gonna get pregnant this month and we won't have to consider anything else but having that baby."

He's good at his professional cheerleading. I can't join in, though. Four years of it all has taken the cheerleader right out of me. And as I look into his eyes, I know that chances are I will have to think about these new alternatives. And I don't want to . . .

"Anybody home?" I call as I open the front door. I'm greeted by a deliriously happy cocker spaniel, and a reclining husband hidden behind the evening newspaper.

"Hey, honey, how'd it go?" he asks without shifting the sports page.

"Okay." I lean over the back of the recliner and kiss him hello between the football scores and the tire advertisements, and then look down at the front page lying in his lap. "Let me see that," I point, and he hands me the rest of the paper. "Did you see this about the latest 'test-tube baby?' " I ask.

"Yeah."

"There's a specialist speaking about in vitro fertilization tonight in town. I'm thinking about going. Want to go with me?" I ask.

"Can't. Remember? I've got that meeting. But you go ahead," he mumbles and goes back to his reading.

I scan a little of the article then look up. "You know, it's absolutely amazing some of the things that medicine is coming up with. I really don't know what I think about them, though. Like this article. What do you think about 'test-tube babies?' "

"Hmmm, nothing much."

"Honey."

He glances over to me. "What?"

"I mean, you know—personally."

"You mean, for us?"

"Well, yeah. Have you ever thought about it?"

"No."

"Well?"

"Well, what?"

I roll my eyes. "What do you think about it?"

He lowers his paper a little and looks at me. "Are you telling me that your doctor has given up on this latest try?"

"No, not really. We were just discussing the new methods a little."

"Well, then, I'll tell you what I think. I think we shouldn't worry about it now." he declares, raising the paper back up. "We'll just jump off that bridge when we come to it."

I start to reply, then give it up. "Okay, then. What's for supper?" I say, in my best sarcastic voice. He lowers the paper and I have his full attention.

At 8:00, I pull up to the college lecture hall, where the meeting is taking place. Wow, I think. Look at all the cars! I hope this is the right place.

Inside, the place is packed. What was I expecting? Whatever it was, it wasn't this. It's standing room only—couples from all walks of life. There's a young executive-type with his designer-clad wife. Sitting by them is a man who looks as if he kicked the farm dirt off his boots, grabbed his wife, jumped in the pick-up and came on in. I see a couple I know from school. I had no idea they were having trouble having another child.

. . . And the biggest surprise of all. I see the man we've come to hear, and he's curly-headed, smiling, and only a little older than I am. He's already fielding questions on in vitro fertilization, explaining how the media has sensationally dubbed it "test-tube babies"—stealing the idea from the book Brave New World*—how there are no test tubes, only a dish in which the fertilization is attempted, and how it is an alternative for some women who, until now, had no alternative at all.*

He is very realistic in his presentation. Actually, he seems almost pessimistic as he discusses how clinics have popped up everywhere— some good, some suspect, and how the success rates in most clinics are dismally low. Then he adds the clincher: each attempt costs several thousand dollars a piece. . . .

Yet hands fly up all over the room.

"What constitutes a possible candidate?" someone asks.

"Where do we sign up?"

"How long is the waiting period?" others chime in.

Unbelievable! *I think.* Thousands of dollars a shot, low odds, and still? . . . I want children, but these people <u>want</u> children.

And then one woman grabs the speaker's attention.

"Doctor," she begins, "I'm no expert or anything, but what about the ethics of all this? What do you think about such things as embryo loss? What about these success rates? And about, well, all those unusual things that can be done with in vitro? Like, say, embryo banking, or surrogate motherhood, or even sex selection?" A low rumbling drifts across the crowd. The woman looks around, a little nervous, then goes on. "Like I say, I'm no expert, but I suppose what I'm asking is, should we do something just because we can? What have you decided about all this?"

The specialist waits for a moment, then answers. "Well, I have settled these issues, personally, a long time ago. And naturally since I'm working with this new method, I am all for it—because of the possible end result. But, I believe strongly that the ethical issue must be decided by you, personally, before you attempt any of the new methods."

Ethical issue? *I think.* "Embryo loss"? "Embryo . . . banking"? What in the world . . .?! "Should we do something just because we can?" she had asked. I haven't even *begun* to think about such things, and I'm not sure I really want to. And I'm not sure I think it's fair to have to.

I stop, though, and examine my heart: How many ways and at what cost will I pursue this baby quest? Is every option modern technology is handing us worthy of trying? Or must I pick and choose— sizing them to fit my ethics?

And for the million dollar question: What are *my ethics on the subject?!*

I don't know. I just want to have a baby . . .

My head is suddenly pounding.

"Any more questions?" *the specialist is asking.*

You bet, *I want to say.* I've got some more:

Will I ever have a child?

What must I go through to have one?

And when—**when**—did my ethics get dragged into the whole frustrating mess?

SHOULD WE CONSIDER THESE NEW ALTERNATIVES?

The Ethical Crisis

Just a few short years ago, this chapter wouldn't have existed. I wouldn't be shoulder-deep in articles and books and opinions and legalities and debates, and we wouldn't have any "alternatives" that needed such moral and legal scrutiny. When the time came to realize that the usual methods of curing infertility were not going to work for us, we'd simply do one of two things—we'd shuffle over to get in line for adoption or we'd make the most of living without children. And that's about it.

But ironically, just when most of the world is wanting fewer and fewer babies, medical science has exploded with answers to make more babies. Answers that give us incredible responsibility. Answers that have the potential to be very, very good, and very, very bad . . .

. . . Answers that can give people like us incredible headaches. Why? We could just jump right in and laud medical science as a savior. Many people do, taking for granted its miracles, blindly embracing its breakthroughs, and then demanding our right to the knowledge.

We could be like the woman who, shortly after the world's first "test-tube" baby was born in England, sued an American hospital because it had stopped an experimental in vitro procedure she had been a part of years before. They had denied her her "rights," she believed. The moment that first "test-tube" baby became a reality, then the technology became her "right."[1]

Or we could be like one person who, when asked about this explosion in biotechnology, said. "Oh, I've read about it, all right. But I've carefully avoided forming any convictions about any of it."

Yet, are either of these responses "right?" Can we afford the luxury of selective consideration because we might benefit from the techniques? In other words—does our own personal set of ethics have anything to do with it all?

You bet it does. It must. The only way it won't is to ignore this part of the infertility crisis in a sort of tunnel vision approach to what we *want*, no matter what the cost. But even that might not work. These alternatives are so packed with questions of one shape or another, that ignoring them may just be asking for trouble later.

So where does that leave us? Right here. Here, wondering exactly what we should know about these new alternatives, here attempting to see both sides of the issues and then here, examining them with a clear head . . . and possibly acquiring that ethical headache in the process.

Sounds pretty heavy, doesn't it? But really, the whole thing boils down to one question: *Should we accept everything that modern biotechnology offers us without question?* We don't hesitate to rely on a cancer or a polio breakthrough, then why do we have qualms about breakthroughs in fertilization techniques?

But we do. And maybe we should. We should certainly not go into it with arms open and eyes closed. To an infertile couple, any infertile couple, that would be the temptation.

As much as it may be against our personal feelings, we must examine the alternatives closely, no matter how nice, how full of hope they sound. We have to examine their worthiness, their acceptability, their ramifications.

The Warnock Inquiry, a British board made up of philosophers, ethicists, lawyers, statesmen, and doctors set up to examine the ethical problems of these new procedures, stated that our society must have "some barriers that are not to be crossed, some limits fixed, beyond which people must not be allowed to go. . . . The very existence of morality depends on it."[2]

The "very existence of morality"? Plainly, these words make it clear we are not dealing with the normal medical accomplishment. We're grappling with something quite different. Not a disease to conquer but a medical boundary to break through—one that may very well change the way we live and think and believe and act. The basic issues are *immensely* bigger than our personal part in them and, as possible participants, we must be aware of them—and we must examine them and all of their ramifications. Our choices are still our choices, but the best sort of choice is the informed one.

What then *are* the basic ethical dilemmas of the new procedures? What about these methods bother the ethicists of our day?

As I began wading through all the material on these new procedures, I wondered what all the fuss was about. And I found out that there is truly much we should look at. In a very sobering sense, we have opened a Pandora's box that will never be shut again.

How complicated can it be? *Very.* The option of *A.I.D.* (*artificial insemination by a donor*) is one way to a baby, but its simplicity covers some hidden, unresolved issues. And, the wonderful possibilities of *I.V.F.* (*in vitro fertilization*) are edged with all the other possibilities it also makes feasible, things we may not think so wonderful. We as couples facing infertility see only the way toward that baby. Others see the threat of abuse of this brave new world technology, all the embryos that are created and never used, all the techniques that are potentially now in our ever-more-powerful hands because of I.V.F. technology—*embryo transfer, sex selection, genetic engineering, embryo banking, surrogate motherhood,* to name only a few. And they wonder, for good reason, whether we are wise enough to handle such power . . .

Where *is* the line drawn? Is it okay to use I.V.F. with a married couple, but not okay to use another's man sperm for the procedure? Is it okay to create several embryos through hyperstimulation of a woman's ovaries in the quest for a higher chance of I.V.F. success, but not to freeze the remaining embryos for another time, or even another couple? Is it okay to use A.I.D., but not its opposite—embryo or egg donor programs?

And that's only the tip of the proverbial iceberg. We as people who could benefit from these new techniques wish them to be simple. But they aren't cooperating. Therefore, we must ferret out the good from the questionable and then ask ourselves if we can accept the good if it makes possible the questionable.

A.I.D., I.V.F. and the *Possibilities with I.V.F.*—these are the three categories the ethical questions seem to fall into. So, let's examine them that way:

A.I.D.—ARTIFICIAL INSEMINATION BY DONOR

You'd think that any procedure that's been around since 1890, used extensively for thirty years and has produced at least 250,000 children, would have all the kinks worked out by now. But by its very nature, the procedure is couched in vagueness, secrecy, and lack of information. One doctor who's performed A.I.D. for most of those thirty years felt a need to do a long-term study on the effects on the children. But he found it impossible. Parents would tell him not to contact them anymore: "We don't want to think of them as inseminated," they would say. "They are our children."[3]

Because of such secrecy, we know very little about what the long-term effects are. Most couples are counseled not to tell the child of his/her unusual origins. And such an action is understandable for the parents making such a long-ranging decision. Yet, is it commendable—or even possible—to keep such a secret? One psychiatrist dealing with A.I.D. plainly declares: "Family secrets are corrosive. You can keep facts secret, but the psychological climate is awful."[4] On the surface, it seems to be a private decision affecting only the parents, but the child soon becomes the focus of concern. One couple sees both sides of the issue very personally:

> The decision to use [A.I.D.] is a lifetime matter. Do we tell the child? . . . [T]he decision to let people know may someday cause our child to ask about his "real" father. On the other hand, can we comfortably live the life? Does our child have the right to know that the father he has known is not his "real" father? . . .

And maybe the most important thought of all:

> . . . If we really do believe we are doing the right thing, why not be open about it?[5]

Many feel that the situation with A.I.D. is reminiscent of adoption only a few years ago, the over-preoccupation with the welfare of the participants at the expense of the child, the fear of the child wanting to find biological parents, and even the sociological stigma of not being totally accepted by everyone. But more than one expert in the field believes that obsessive concern with self-protection needs to give way to concern for the child. Many of the ethical exceptions experts take with the new alternatives center around the welfare of the child being created, and the absence of enough restrictions, guidelines, or concern for this possible new human being.

Yet, none of the issues is so much in the hands of the parents as the decision to tell the A.I.D. child of his/her conception. Should the child be told or not? A couple who has opted for A.I.D. due to genetic reasons, such as hemophilia, may find telling their child about A.I.D. somewhat easier—and even wise. The child, in essence, does not have to worry about acquiring the father's disorder. Other couples may not find it so easy. And, in fact, the vast majority still opt for secrecy. Not telling means a commitment to keeping a lifelong secret.

But the news may still slip. One study of A.I.D. children found that the few children who were told anything were told in a punitive way. In one situation, for instance, the husband, mad at his wife, turned to their child and said, "I'm not really your father."[6] A French study found that nearly half of those who initially intended to keep it a secret told someone. And we know too well that the moment that happens, our control over the information is gone.

Lori Andrews, in a *Psychology Today* article, tells of one A.I.D. child who found out when she was thirteen. By that time, the girl's mother had divorced her first husband, the man she was married to when she was artificially inseminated. The girl had a normal father/daughter relationship with him, but had a strained relationship with her mother's new husband, her stepfather. One day, as the teenager packed to visit her "real" father, her stepfather exploded with the news: "He's no more your father than I am!"

Another woman, who found out her dad was not her biological father when she was thirty-one felt her life had been "some sort of fiction." She said, "I want to know my background, my medical history, but I also want to know precisely what he had in mind when he was a donor. . . . Didn't he feel any type of concern? My parents had an unhappy marriage. Didn't he feel any sort of responsibility for the life he was creating?"[7] And with that, she began her search to find him and ask him.

"Many of the children of artificial insemination feel used," states Emma May Vilarid, who in 1974 founded an organization called the International Soundex Reunion Registry to match, without charge, children and their biological parents they have never met. "They feel that half of their heritage is missing. They feel they have a right to recorded genetic information."[8] But just as in adoption, some children don't react negatively at all to such news. Why would A.I.D. children respond so unpredictably to the same fact of life? Maybe the answer lies in the possibility that children respond to how their parents act about such facts.

The decision to tell or not to tell is an integral one to the decision to go through the A.I.D. alternative. And the way we *feel* about that decision *will* have long-ranging effects, effects we may not be prepared for because we may have rushed into those decisions. Rushing into this hopeful step in our baby quest may keep us from the heavy thinking we need to give it. Doctors may ignore the emotions involved with A.I.D. as they go about giving us what we want. Innocently, the doctor might unveil the news of a husband's infertility in one breath, and in the next explain that the wife can still have a baby by using another man's sperm. If the ticking of that biological clock forces you to hurry with this decision, anything could happen, because emotions are so intimately involved. One awful example is of the man who initially agreed to A.I.D. but later changed his mind and convinced his wife, by then pregnant through A.I.D., to have an abortion. Yet, four years later after he had accepted his infertility, they went through A.I.D. again and conceived.[9]

The husband's feelings are of utmost importance in this decision. Some men seem to work through it all and decide that having a child is the important thing, an essential part of their life's fulfillment. Others, along with their wives may realize that having a child is not the essential component for a fulfilling life that they have been led to believe. And still others would feel more comfortable with adoption. The tension here is the one with any step in the infertility maze: attempting to keep the marital lines open and flexible, attempting to keep the pespective broad and healthy, attempting to understand and come to terms with what the other partner is feeling. And if the attempt is not successful, that's when it is clear how drastically these new alternatives in specific, and infertility in general, can affect the marital relationship.

Well, then, should prospective A.I.D. parents—or for that matter prospective in vitro and embryo transfer parents—be screened to force self-evaluation or to prove their parental fitness, as they must be with adoption? The problem, of course, is the same one as for adoption. Who decides? Psychologists have become the "gatekeepers" for the more involved alternatives, playing a vital part. One psychologist stated it this way: "It is paramount to identify those couples whose wish for a child masks a chronically troubled relationship or those with less stable coping mechanisms who might not tolerate well the stress and uncertainty inherent in such a program."[10]

A bill proposed in Michigan would require that a marriage counselor, psychologist, or psychiatrist counsel couples who wish to use A.I.D. egg donation, embryo transfer, surrogate motherhood, or embryo freezing, and certify they understand the responsibilities of parenting.

But David Berger, a psychiatrist at University of Toronto's Medical School doesn't like that idea. In working with this very situation over a period of time, he concludes, "I try not to be a judge when interviewing people who wish to use artificial insemination. A lot of people have children without being judged."[11] "It's not my place to pass judgment on these couples," explains Dr. Jose Pliego, infertility specialist at Texas' Scott and White Hospital. "Sure, I want the best situation possible for this child, but I can't push my standards on them. We [doctors] are pro-life, and would like to help our patients accomplish their goals. And that's the level we must deal with them."

So it's that same old tension that drives us crazy, the one we feel when we see a mother yelling at her dirty child on the street corner. Life isn't fair. Some of the people who'd make great parents never get the chance. Some who should never parent, get the chance over and over. But would it be any fairer if there were some human hand making the decisions? Maybe, maybe not. As it is now, the examination is mostly self-examination, left up to the individual couple.

What about examination of the donor, his medical and genetic background? One observer quipped that whatever it is, it's better checked out than the husband's ever was. The warped logic of that aside, this is one of the biggest worries the potential A.I.D. couple will have—and rightly so. Yes, the donor is better "checked out" than the husband, but the couple, being forced to consider having a child another way than with the husband, deserve the best from modern medicine. As theologian G. R. Dunstan stated at an English conference on the subject, doctors should use "higher criteria than those provided by natural random forces."[12] And that is especially true when the couple is contemplating A.I.D. to avoid such genetic disorders as hemophilia, sickle-cell anemia, cystic fibrosis, or Tay-Sachs syndrome (a degenerative disease that affects Jewish children). Looking at the current A.I.D. situation from that mindset, A.I.D.'s donor examination can be lacking. Most doctors will be as conscientious as possible about picking the best donor, but, except in areas close to sperm banks, logistics usually narrow their choices to those available.

Studies show that eighty percent of all donors are medical students. And most often, doctors rely on the honesty of these donors when they fill in information about personal medical background.[13] Besides their availability, doctors also see medical students as good risks because they work with them enough to know them, seeing them overall as intelligent, well-balanced, and healthy. And honest. (The fact that the donor is paid, though, can always bring such honesty into question, no matter who or what he happens to be. . . . The force of that idea shows up seriously in the alternative of surrogating discussed later. Maybe we should take a cue from the British whose donors are truly "donors." They don't get paid.[14])

But even honesty may not be enough. These student donors may not *know* they are carriers of viruses or infections or even recessive genetic disorders. The American Association of Tissue Banks' Reproductive Council is concerned about sperm banking for this reason. Its guidelines point out that one in 150 of the population has a chromosomal abnormality.[15]

A.I.D.'s superficiality of donor screening may cause big problems, for your health and for the baby's. It has happened. As Lori Andrews puts it in her book *New Conceptions:* "It is ironic that the screening of donor sperm for human A.I.D. is much less stringent than that of bull sperm in the cattle industry."[16] And she goes on to quote a research report done on 379 A.I.D. practitioners responsible for 3,576 A.I.D. births that concluded that the screening of donors for genetic diseases is inadequate.

What, then, can you do? The potential A.I.D. couple can ask for and pay for tests to be run on the prospective donor for some chromosome disorders. But that possibility may not be offered routinely. So this may be another time when you must take the initiative—and ask. The money and effort may be worth it for peace of mind—and for health, because the dearth of record-keeping and the habit of destroying records shortly after the procedure will make backtracking in the event of any problem almost impossible.[17]

And that brings up the issue of A.I.D. record-keeping—or lack of it. In most cases, records are either not kept or only kept for a short time. In actuality, then, there is no way to know whether sperm is defective or not. And even stranger, there are no guidelines as to how many times a donor can be used. In some programs, donors are limited to two or three births. Many clinics draw the line at ten. But with the lack of clear guidelines, a donor could be used once or thirty times, never thinking of future involvement.

Whether he wants to or not, however, the donor may be forced to think about that involvement of long ago, as in the case of Dr. Peter Forbes, a California gynecologist. While a medical student in Washington D.C. three decades ago, Forbes provided sperm for thirty-three A.I.D. pregnancies. Realizing now that one of his "children" could theoretically prove his paternity, Forbes amended his will to state that any child not borne of his wife will be entitled to only one dollar from his estate.

And because of such lack of clear-cut guidelines, there is a possibility, however remote, of unwitting incest. A few doctors have already stopped weddings between children who shared the same donor. In fact, Forbes has said that if he knew any of his "children," who would now be in their twenties, he would tell them: "Don't marry anyone from D.C."[18]

And the obvious possibility for single people to take advantage of this technology cannot be overlooked, even though so far there seems to be an unspoken guideline with most programs that the procedures will be open only to married couples. But unspoken guidelines or no, there needs to be some legal guidelines, for even if we can accept singles having children (since our society has come to accept their adopting), the idea could allow lesbian couples to view the procedure as a way to have a family—as they are already doing in some areas of the country. As such scenarios make their way to the courts, we'll hopefully see the legal community wake up to this need.

Anything seems possible in this eyebrow-raising time we live in. Home insemination kits are now available. Even choosing a donor is not necessarily a thing only done through doctors. Some intrepid souls are actually taking matters into their own hands. As one woman explained:

> A doctor was the last person I would have gone to to find a donor. Reproduction is a very serious thing. We didn't want to give the responsibility to anyone else. I was not going to carry a child of unknown parentage.[19]

So several of their friends offered to donate sperm. The couple picked one whose wife they knew could handle the idea and drew up a contract detailing everybody's rights.

This is where the matter gets truly complicated and where we may begin to wonder how such openness will affect the family. If things keep going the way they seem to be, the idea of family may have to be redefined. Just like a family that includes a bunch of ex-spouses, and stepchildren and half-siblings, A.I.D. families may begin to—may be forced to—include biological parents too. The term "extended family" has been tacked on this sort of possibility. Many psychologists predict that the norm *will* be for the A.I.D. child of the future to know about his or her biological family—a scenario in which the donor will be known and will stay in contact with the couple and the child. And such a scenario could include surrogate mothers as well.

One sperm bank in California allows sperm donors to list their names and addresses to be made available to the child at age eighteen. Another proposed Michigan law would make it mandatory that such information as name and medical history of any donor—be it sperm, egg, embryo, or womb—be made available to the child at eighteen. One man is allowing the release of his name and intends to design a portfolio about himself to give to the child. And he says he's even willing to paticipate in the parenting process. As he puts it, "I imagine it would develop along the lines of the role a divorced father takes."[20]

And if that isn't startling enough, there have also been donors who've gone to court to establish visitation rights to the children they helped to create. The lawyer for one mother explained what he considered to be the legal and the sociological problem with such a situation:

> The court is trying to force the creation of a family. . . . It's hard enough for people to get along with their ex–husbands or ex–wives in order to bring up a child decently, let alone to impose that upon two people who have never had any relationship whatsoever.[21]

And therein lies the problem. In his book *Brave New People*, D. Gareth Jones brings up the concept that even though A.I.D. has its good uses, they can't keep him from worrying about its effect on the basic unity of marriage. He speaks of the unknown result of A.I.D.'s break in a couple's "biological bond." And he may be touching on a subtle A.I.D. problem. Although the use of A.I.D. can come from the highest expression of love, it can, in a very real way, raise our reproductive capacity above everything, making the need for a baby so integral to marital unity that a foreign element is brought into the couple's most intimate circle. And from what we see of the instances above, such a break in a couple's biological unity just might have a ripple effect on the family unity that the couple has risked so much to have.

Whether any of the above could happen to us if we chose A.I.D. is something we cannot foresee. And there are large numbers of people who believe that the potential pitfalls of A.I.D. can be avoided through sensitive counseling and the highest participation possible by the husband in the insemination process (some going so far as to not only be there, but to actually do the insemination under the guidance of the doctor).

And maybe this new sort of extended family that looks so scary won't be any more of a problem than the situation we already have of adopted children finding and befriending their biological parents, and the one of divorced fathers and stepparents and various types of blending families. We seem to have accepted such unusual arrangements so far. The question probably should be whether such blendings are healthy or hurtful, especially when our decisions give us control over the possibility of such blendings.

There's no doubt that more legal guidelines can alleviate many of the grey areas. The call from most authorities is for some action from the court, maybe involving sealed documents only opened after the child is an adult, for instance. A.I.D., however, is too multifaceted not to have some of its current practices called into question, practices that many participants will find advantageous and safe and will want to keep, such as donor anonymity, payment, and lack of record-keeping. And yet, for the sake of the child being created, some of these risks must be taken so that protective guidelines can be set not just for the participants, but for the creation. And as long as the legal aspects of A.I.D. remain in the twilight zone, they cannot help anyone.

THE RELIGIOUS ISSUE

Are there specifically religious problems posed by A.I.D.? The Roman Catholic church considers A.I.D. adultery and the child illegitimate. Orthodox Judaism has, overall, also taken a firm position against A.I.D., while Reform Judaism seems more open to it.[22] As for Protestant Christian denominations, the Lutheran Church has come out against it, but most of the rest are either divided or leave it up to the individual believer and his/her own conviction, even though there are some leaders who are adamant in their denunciation of it.

Is A.I.D. a sort of long-distance adultery? An exaggeration of the idea of a break in "biological bond?"

From a psychological viewpoint, if not a religious one, to say such a thing is not to understand the plight, the mindset of the infertile couple. The woman can easily feel the pressure and guilt of such thinking, but as we understand adultery, it calls for a "breach of faith," as one writer explained it.[23] And there is no breach of faith between an A.I.D. couple. Rather, the opposite is usually the case when a well-thought-out decision is made to use A.I.D. One woman who experienced A.I.D. described her husband as more committed to having a child than most of her friend's husbands because he willingly committed himself to love a child that wasn't going to be his biologically. As she so aptly put it, "He gave so much more than one night of sex."[24]

The diversity in religious thought on A.I.D. as well as on the other alternatives, is unbelievable. Some seem to think in vitro (I.V.F.) is all right, since it is using medicine to the utmost for the husband/wife relationship. Others will say that A.I.D. is quite acceptable, but that in vitro fertilization is suspect.

Henlee Barnette, professor emeritus of Christian Ethics at Southern Baptist Theological Seminary, and Clinical Professor

of Psychiatry and Behaviorial Sciences at University of Louis-
ville School of Medicine, suggests a more open mind toward
I.V.F.:

> Some argue that in vitro fertilization is not God's plan of re-
> production. . . . The only legitimate mode of reproducing, it is
> argued, is coital. But where this is impossible in some females,
> are they to be deprived of children of their own when the means
> for conception and full-term delivery are available?

And on the adultery issue, he adds: "Some churchmen equate
the 'means' with adultery, but how can this be so when there
is no sex act, no passion, no lust?"[25]

Yet some would disagree, feeling that masturbation, no matter what the circumstance, is an issue, whether in I.V.F. or
A.I.D. Dr. Robert Wells, a doctor who deals with the study and
treatment of infertility and who performed A.I.D. for years,
now goes on record as believing it to be wrong, because ". . .
lust is built into the technique of donor artificial insemination
when one honestly takes into account the methods donors
must use to collect their sperm specimens."[26]

Gareth Jones poses a problem with A.I.D. that speaks to us
on a different, more personal level:

> More profoundly, A.I.D. may be a manifestation of a couple's
> unwillingness to share a common fate, that of being unable to
> bear a child. . . . Sharing in this instance would amount to fore-
> going having a child or, alternatively, having a child by adoption.
> Either of these options would circumvent the possibility of a bro-
> ken marital relationship, and may amount to the truest expression
> of love for one's neighbor.[27]

Though this idea may at first sound stark, he may have
caught an essential point worthy of consideration by any couple. It makes us go back to the core of what marriage is, what
marriage is structured to be, especially from a religious point
of view. Is it to have babies? I don't think so. The world is
replenished. Still, the yearning to procreate is built-in, all right,
and there's no surgery that can undo it. But Jones has some-

thing to say we should hear, even if we have a passel of kids. In explaining that enormous care must be taken in deciding for or against A.I.D., he expresses ideas we might wish to ignore but cannot:

> . . . We should not accept the view that human beings can do anything we wish, and can solve all problems confronting them. Perhaps one of the supreme virtues is the ability, on occasions, to accept loss, inadequacy and suffering. It is well known that marriages can be very successful even in the absence of children, although most would regard such marriages as deficient in a desirable element.[28]

As you can see, there is much complexity to this simple A.I.D. procedure, and enough confusion to merit an in-depth look. A.I.D. may pose too many questions for you to consider. The donor idea alone may have too many question marks attached for you to consider the option.

But however you feel right now, you will probably be offered it as an alternative if your infertility work-up goes far enough. Concerned specialists who are striving to find an answer that will make everyone happy view A.I.D. as a very acceptable alternative. It is "pro-life," as many doctors would put it, and it is an answer, one being used on a wider scale than you might have ever imagined. But doctors cannot give you the whole picture because they don't deal with the whole picture. And very little study has been done on that whole picture due to A.I.D.'s secretive nature. Yet you desperately need to know as much as you can about it, because the real problems come when a couple doesn't carefully and honestly work through their feelings about this life-long decision.

IN VITRO FERTILIZATION

Legally and ethically, I.V.F. (in vitro fertilization) is in a state of flux. Legally, I.V.F. and the rights of I.V.F. patients are, as medical law expert Lori Andrews puts it, "a current crazy quilt of state laws."[29] And the result is a hazy legal situation. State rather than federal laws govern the relationship between you and your doctor, so each state decides its own medical parameters. And that leaves the door open to two sorts of laws concerning I.V.F.: (1) those that were on the books before I.V.F. was developed yet, by their language, seem to cover it, and (2) those that were passed with I.V.F. in mind.

Some states have fetal research laws that inhibit doctors opening I.V.F. clinics. In Minnesota, for instance, law forbids experimentation (and in most ways, I.V.F. is still considered experimental) on an embryo unless the experiment protects its health or life, or scientific evidence exists that shows the experiment to be harmless. In Massachusetts the law has been interpreted to mean that I.V.F. would not violate their state's fetal research law if all the fertilized eggs were implanted in the woman. An 1877 Illinois law that makes the doctor criminally liable if he or she endangers the life or health of an embryo obviously affects the state's idea of today's I.V.F. biotechnology. The law doesn't outlaw I.V.F, but it plants enough apprehension in the minds of the state's doctors that no one will attempt it. Also, as it stands now, the Illinois I.V.F. doctor would also be granted custody of the child, but the law never arranges for the parents to regain custody.[30]

So, the legal situation concerning I.V.F. is a mess. And although calls are being made to create some sort of semblance of unified national order out of it all, the law changes slowly—either way—for or against, as witnessed with A.I.D.

The ethical arguments swirling around I.V.F, though, are more easily defined and easily stated than with A.I.D.—if not more easily resolved. The need for concern is real, and looming larger every day. The American Fertility Society in 1985 established an ethics committee to investigate for itself these new reproductive technologies. An Ethics Advisory Board was set up by the Department of Health, Education, and Welfare as early as 1979 to decide whether I.V.F. was ethically acceptable. In deciding that it was, the Board members went on to be very specific that the term "ethically acceptable" would be defined as "ethically defensible," and *not* necessarily "ethically right."[31]

That, in essence, puts the decision whether I.V.F. is "ethically right" back in our individual laps. And that decision must call up many questions: Are we playing God? Tampering with nature? What is the status of the embryo? Is it a person or is it property? Should it have the full rights of personhood at conception? If so, should we take into consideration how many are unavoidably lost in the process? What should be done with these spare embryos? Is it unethical to include a fetus in an experimental procedure when it cannot consent and might be harmed? Should we create possible life if we don't intend immediately to give it the chance to live, as in the case of using embryos for research? Is infertility truly a medical need? Or is it a desire? And should we be doctoring desires? It's enough to make your head swim, but these are the very real, very timely ethical concerns.

But those are only the ones concerning I.V.F. specifically. What about all the consequences of I.V.F., that Pandora's box of futuristic biotechnical applications? Will something good cause the possibility of something bad? Can we accept I.V.F. if we do not accept what it makes possible? Tampering with nature, the status of the embryo, fetal harm, embryo loss, the medical mandate for I.V.F., and all those futuristic possibilities. . . . These are the major issues. Let's look at them closely.

TAMPERING WITH NATURE?

Playing God. That's the way we hear this issue expressed the most. . . . Are we tampering with the natural laws? Are we going too far in our medical "miracles"? These questions finally lead to the one big question that will be answered in the near future, one way or another: "Is there a place for the new biotechnology within the balance of nature?" There seems to be three trains of thought on the place of I.V.F. and its possibilities in our world.

We could give a blanket "no" to that question, as many people do, believing that in vitro fertilization is "unnatural." Such people are worried that we are playing with fire, getting into areas we were never meant to go, taking on responsibilities we cannot handle and were never made to handle. Playing God. These people, especially many within the religious community, will find *all* the biotechnical "miracles" off limits. Anything not absolutely nature's way of reproducing, even including A.I.H., artificial insemination by husband, is wrong.

We could give a blanket "yes," not seeing anything wrong but seeing everything right with the breakthroughs and experimentations of the new biotechnology. The ethical problem would, then, not exist.

Or third, as opposed to saying a blanket "yes" or a blanket "no," we would answer a calm "yes"—with stipulations. Religious ethicists who hold this view see such medical breakthroughs from the perspective that God has called us to be cocreators, to take serious responsibility in uncovering nature's secrets. Such thinking would call upon us to take an active part in all these new technologies. We would be bringing our morality and our ethics to these alternatives, giving them moral parameters and then taking full responsibility for how we are improving on Mother Nature's design, and how we lovingly help people overcome defects not of their own making.

So the argument boils down to these three trains of thought. If you believe that we are called to use our talents ethically in uncovering nature's secrets and working toward a better world, then you will embrace the new technology and see these breakthroughs as godsends. You may study I.V.F. and decide that although all the steps of the procedures—taking the sperm and the egg and placing them into a dish—seem terribly manipulative and humanly plotted, the important things are still intact from that point on.

But if you believe we are tampering with nature, playing God, then you will pull back from I.V.F., and you'll worry that in tampering with the natural way, we are courting disaster. You'd have to decide what exactly tampering with nature is, though. As Dr. Howard Jones, the American I.V.F. pioneer, points out:

> Actually, every request of a physician to diagnose and treat disease is a request to manipulate nature. If it is ethically acceptable to seek medical care for a reproductive disorder, it is ethically acceptable to seek care that requires in vitro fertilization.[32]

According to Dr. Jones, then, we have been tampering with nature since medicine began. Yet there is still that scary idea of crossing over into a no-man's land of human procreation. Maybe this sort of tampering is different, we may think. And that may cause enough concern to question our participation in any of the new procedures. For those of us dealing with the ethical question in a personal way, maybe that personal answer can come through a specific study of I.V.F.'s other controversial issues:

STATUS OF THE EMBRYO

Is the embryo a person or is it property? If this debate sounds vaguely familiar, it's because it hits squarely on the abortion issue, where this question has had its effects as well. The case of the orphaned frozen embryos in Australia, brings this issue into focus. (As discussed in Section 3, the embryos were orphaned when an American woman tried I.V.F. there, having her extra embryos frozen and stored, but then died with her husband in a plane crash before anything was decided about her embryos.) The embryos were filed in cold storage in 1981 because no one could decide one fundamental question: Does every embryo have the right to a womb? If so, then what about Roe vs. Wade, the Supreme Court decision allowing abortion that has been read to mean that a fetus has no right to life? If that's so, then the embryos could be destroyed.

But nobody's doing it. An Australian ethics board set up to decide their fate suggested they be destroyed. But Australian lawmakers voted, instead, to recommend they be given a chance at life through surrogate wombs. Still, the question remains. As a *Newsweek* article put it:

> At what point, if any, after conception, does an unborn being possess legal rights? If anti-abortion forces could manage to establish that a frozen embryo has a right to a womb, the notion of abortion on demand might be mortally wounded.[33]

What is the status of the embryo? When does it become a person worthy of protection? At conception? At implantation, six to ten days? At transition to a fetus at eight weeks? At "quickening," about twenty weeks? At birth? Both issues, abortion and I.V.F., are deeply affected by this one quandary.

I.V.F. forces us to ask questions, though. What is the embryo's status, morally and biologically? Can we view it as morally acceptable to use them in "clinical I.V.F." (the term for using embryos for creating life in a mother's womb), and not to use them in "laboratory I.V.F." (the term for using embryos for purely experimental purposes)? If we believe the embryo contains the "soul," or even if we feel it deserves our respect as a potential "soul," can we allow one and not the other?

Dr. Jones believes there is no way to know when the "ensoulment," the moment when the soul enters the embryo, begins. In his view, to say that the embryo is the beginning of life is to say that what made that embryo, the sperm and the egg, were not alive. And he also points out that fertilization does not necessarily result in a human individual. In one type of twinning (when twins form), the formation of the two embryos doesn't occur until much later, and in some instances fertilization can result not in an embryo, but in a tumor.[34]

Princeton Seminary's Paul Ramsey, one of the U.S.'s leading medical ethicists, has stated that the embryo's "blastocyst" stage is when fetal life should be given protection. That's when the embryo is about sixty to one hundred cells and pulls away from the rest of the mass proving itself not a twin or a tumor. That could be when the first origins of *individual* human life could be established, and, in Ramsey's opinion, when that individual life begins to be inviolate. But he goes on to say that it is relatively unimportant to establish at what point a fetus (or with this train of thought, an embryo) becomes a human, since God values all humans, no matter what stage of development they happen to be.[35]

Roman Catholics, staying true to Pope Pius XII's arguments (that have been interpreted to be against I.V.F. because it is not natural conception), believe the embryo deserves respect as a new human from the time of fertilization.[36] One Catholic moral theologian, though, has broken with Catholic tradition and voiced a new opinion. As part of HEW'S Ethics Advisory Board, Richard McCormick, S.J. came to understand that there were three possible positions on human life at this stage: (1) that an embryo is simply disposable maternal tissue, (2) that an embryo is a human being meriting the protection given to all humans, or (3) that the embryo is a living being, demanding respect, but not yet meriting the full range of personal rights. And as he evaluated what he learned of nature's normal interaction with embryos, McCormick came to his tradition-breaking conclusion:

> I believe that there are serious reasons of a physiologic nature for evaluating the embryo before implantation differently from the embryo that has implanted, or from the newborn. At least 50% of fertilized ova never implant.[37]

Still, the Board, as well as McCormick, made a special point to stress the need to show "respect" for the newly-formed embryo, no matter what its status.

So we are back where we started, with no concrete answers. The embryo, though, does deserve special status in I.V.F. As Colin Honey, a British theologian explains, "It is human life in the sense that nothing essential need be added in the normal process to bring it to maturity. . . ."[38] And he underscores that it deserves special status, if for no other reason than it is not accidentally created.

The law needs to make some decisions to help decide the

status of the embryo. But the issue's overlapping of the abortion issue could easily be impeding any positive address of the issue. The Supreme Court went out of its way to avoid a general ruling on "when life begins." If legislation is passed to define conception as the beginning of life, the abortion issue would be in chaos, and even contraceptive techniques such as IUDs which keep the embryos from implanting, would be affected.[39] As Honey put it, "It may equally be the case . . . that in I.V.F. . . . we will come to see more clearly that practices previously found acceptable are morally repugnant."[40]

FETAL HARM

This issue entails the idea that a fetus cannot consent to be part of I.V.F., so it is unethical to include it in the experiment as long as there is any possibility of harm. A being should not be brought into existence if there is any possibility of damage from the procedure. Biologist and ethicist Leon Kass has argued, "One cannot ethically choose for [the new being] the unknown hazards he must face and simultaneously choose to give him life in which to face them."[41]

In nature, through the high "natural abortion" (miscarriage) rate and through the survival-of-the-fittest ordeal that sperm must go through to fertilize the egg, malformed or weak embryos either never are created or miscarry. If we bypass this natural obstacle course, are we allowing some abnormal embryos to make it that nature would have winnowed out? And if so, who then is responsible for those malformed beings? This is the issue Kass is worried about.

But so far, we have no way of knowing if I.V.F. offers more harm than normal conception. And on the contrary, it's even possible it may cause less damage to the fetus. As mentioned before, very few I.V.F. babies have been born with a defect, and most usually with only cardiac malformation easily corrected by surgery. Thus, time hasn't proven this issue to be of primary concern . . . *yet*. (Some critics would point to the possible practice by some I.V.F. clinics of requiring the mother to sign a consent form for the fetus to be aborted if abnormalities are discovered.[42] In such cases, the I.V.F. practitioners would be making *sure* that the abnormality percentage is acceptably low. Because we truly do not know how much such policies affect the good I.V.F. record, we cannot pass judgment until we do.)

EMBRYO LOSS/SPARE EMBRYOS

If we conclude that the embryo should be respected, then that brings us to the problem of *embryo loss*, another major ethical problem with I.V.F. In nature, embryo loss is very high. And to most ethicists, if the risks are no greater than those found in nature, then I.V.F. is acceptable.

But what about all those embryos that were created during the early stages of I.V.F. research, created specifically to be used in that research? In vitro has a history of very high embryonic death.[43] If embryo loss creates very much of an ethical problem for the infertile couple, they cannot ignore this part of I.V.F.'s history—how we got where we are.

Creating extra embryos is an accepted part of the I.V.F. procedure. To gain the best possibility for success in I.V.F., superovulation is produced . . . that is, you would be given an ovary-stimulating drug such as Clomid or Pergonal to produce as many eggs as possible. What if more than one become fertilized? What do you do with the extra embryos? Clifford Grobstein summed up the ethical dilemma this way: "If it is moral to remove a human egg from a woman and fertilize it (some believe it to be immoral), is it any less moral to do anything more to the subsequent early embryo other than to reinsert it into the uterus of its donor?"[44]

Quite a few answers can be given to that question. In reality, there are three things that can happen to *spare embryos:*

1. They can be put back into the mother's womb and all given a chance for life immediately.

2. They can be used for experimentation.
3. They can be stored, frozen for future use by the woman in later I.V.F. attempts, or used by others in a sort of embryo adoption.

American I.V.F. specialists have for the most part believed that the most moral thing to do is put all the embryos in the woman's womb. But that practice, of course, could cause multiple births and multiple hazards to the pregnancy. Some medical soul-searching is now being done on this point. Dr. Gary Hodgen, the scientific director of the Jones Institute of Reproductive Medicine in Norfolk, has said that many groups are deciding that it's unethical to transfer more than three embryos. "If [the doctor] puts six fresh embryos in the uterus at the same time," he explains, "the problem is the multiple pregnancy rate . . . rises to 28%. . . ."[45] And that is not a percentage to ignore. The impact of such multiple pregnancies, these doctors believe, on the wellbeing of the mother, fetus, and family cannot be ignored any longer.

And there's another catch. Nobody can predict how many eggs will be created by I.V.F.'s hyperstimulation of a woman's ovaries. For instance, one clinic in Dallas retrieved ten eggs from one woman, and nine of them fertilized and were transferable. The doctor implanted six, the normal maximum. So the question then was what to do with the extra embryos? After the Dallas I.V.F. specialist searched in vain for a woman in midcycle who might "adopt" the embryos, he was forced to destroy them.[46]

What about embryo freezing? Almost 200 human embryos, known only by their mother's name, have been held in a frozen state of suspended animation in Melbourne, Australia. Australians have allowed spare embryos to be adopted, and one Briton involved with the procedure has said that the only ethical thing to do is freeze them.

But the idea of *embryo storage banks* makes quite a lot of people nervous. The British Medical Association Ethics Committee warned, "Medical technology is running ahead of morality," and would rather see a moratorium put on storage banks until study can be done.[47] That, of course, may not stop further experimentation. State officials in Australia accuse the I.V.F. clinic involved with the orphaned frozen embryos of "thumbing its nose" at the government by pushing onward with I.V.F. technology. And one doctor who recently quit the fertilization team said: "This is a perfect example of the processes being used before there has been a chance to think through the problems."[48]

Dr. Hodgen believes he has one answer, an answer that's already been successfully used. He suggests that storing unfertilized eggs might be more acceptable: "Freezing eggs is better than freezing embryos that some people already consider members of the population."[49]

As for using embryos for experimental purposes, scientists such as I.V.F. pioneers Steptoe and Edwards believe spare embryos can be very useful, teaching us about early human life and helping us to insure normality in I.V.F. babies. Using spare embryos for experimental purposes could in theory help us overcome genetic diseases, such as cystic fibrosis, sickle-cell anemia, schizophrenia, even perhaps cancer, saving thousands and thousands of lives. Yet is it moral to create potential life just to experiment with it? Even in the name of common good? Maybe more fairly, this is a question that should have been posed during the years leading up to the first I.V.F., before the very first embryo was created to be studied and destroyed.

What then is the ethical answer for what we should do with these spare embryos? We could abstain from creating those extra embryos in the first place, attempting I.V.F. with the usual single egg a woman creates in a given month. But that would cut an already low I.V.F. success rate down to as low as five percent.[50] No couple choosing to go through the grueling rigors of I.V.F., paying the high price tag for each try, wants to hear such an answer. But even more realistically, it is not an answer that most I.V.F. practitioner/researchers would want to entertain for a moment. These embryos are too important to the well-being of the I.V.F. programs as a whole.

And this whole line of thinking seems to me to raise the question of motives. . . . When I listen objectively, I can't help but wonder what is actually at the heart of all this biotechnical energy. Is it truly an effort to help the infertile couple? Or . . . is the real issue the idea of pushing ahead the boundaries of modern medical expertise? That thought may be what troubles me most.

As in most cases where humans are involved, the two aspects probably are intertwined. But there is still that idea of moral responsibility. Why aren't the low success rates more openly discussed and written about? The misleading vagueness of success rate guidelines discussed in Section 3 can't be ignored. In vitro is still very experimental in many, many ways, and the procedure should be more honestly portrayed. Why isn't it? Does the possibility that such honesty might lower the number of couples vying to be experimental patients have anything to do with it? If the good of the patient is uppermost, why hasn't everyone pooled their resources toward the end of better technique?

As Honey asks, what about compassion mixed with apparent ethical considerations involved?

> Is it more loving to admit an infertile woman to a difficult programme with perhaps less than 10% chance of a pregnancy in her case than to counsel adoption or some other course? . . . If for example, face lifts only worked in 10–20% of cases—and in the remainder the patient's face returned to the original wrinkled condition I suspect that doctors would be reluctant to perform them, no matter how keenly they were desired. Even the small risk associated with general anaesthetic would assume greater proportions.[51]

Likening infertility to face lifts seems a little trivializing, but in the sense that the patient is at risk for a very low percentage chance of getting what she went "under the knife" for, the idea has merit. The doctors may believe we have the right to assume that risk if we choose to. Many infertile couples will do just that, and do so gladly (even, as Leon Kass would protest taking the risk for the potential fetus, too). But what may have the most merit is the possibility that medical science, if however innocently, may be taking advantage of the infertile patients' very real desperation, a desperation that would see any chance as a good chance.

MEDICAL MANDATE—DOCTORING DESIRES?

This debate centers around the question of whether infertility is a real medical need, and whether I.V.F. is actually a medical treatment, since it does nothing for a couples' infertility problem, bypassing it altogether.

These sort of debates seem irrelevant for anyone going through the infertility grind. We would probably agree with England's Warnock Inquiry that sees medicine as also doctoring physical malfunctions. And infertility could be seen as that— not a life-threatening malfunction, but one like cataracts, the removal of which would aid the quality of life.

The concept of desire vs. need, though, is one we all should think about, because it does have its ramifications. Ethicist Paul Ramsey believes we are doctoring desires, and, as he explains it, if we begin to do that, where will we stop?

> . . . [I]f medicine turns to doctoring desires instead of medical conditions, if medicine provides a woman with a child without actually curing her infertility, is there any reason for doctors to be reluctant to accede to parents' desires to have a girl rather than a boy, blonde hair rather than brown, a genius rather than a clout . . . or alternatively a child who because of his idiosyncrasies would have a good career as a freak in a circus?[52]

And such an outlandish look at how we might go too far introduces the next problem many people have with I.V.F.— what I.V.F. *allows.* Ramsey's genetic engineering idea is only one of the things let loose by opening I.V.F.'s Pandora's box of possibilities.

THE STARTLING POSSIBILITIES FOR THE FUTURE—AND NOW

"Embryo stores," "Fertilizers," "Social Predestinators"— these words from *Brave New World,* unquestionably science fiction terms a few years ago, sound chillingly current now. It's amazing to think how quickly we've been ushered into the presence of these futuristic possibilities. In 1970, when Alvin Toffler foretold the coming of such biological technology as buying embryos, genetic engineering, and other forms of what he called "birth technology" in his landmark book *Future Shock,* the concepts sounded too amazing for us to ever experience in our lifetime. But many of the projections are already possible. The others are waiting in the wings. And the majority of them will be made possible through I.V.F. technology.

The possibilities with I.V.F. technology touch the nerve of modern responsibility. Slowly we are realizing we can't ignore what the technology can be used for. One religious ethicist has said I.V.F. may not be immoral, but it *is* "morally risky."[53] That idea, as we've seen, is heavily debated. But few would deny that I.V.F.'s *possibilities* are morally risky. To say the very least. What *can* we do with all this knowledge? The answers are mind-boggling.

The problem of Australia's orphaned frozen embryos is only the beginning. As the head of the President's Commission on Medical Ethics commented about that situation: "The notion that you can have a child born years and years after the death of his parents is something completely new. . . . This case is a kind of beacon indicating that we have trouble ahead."[54]

And what about the young widow in France whose husband had frozen his sperm before he died of cancer? She wanted to bear his child, but when she asked for his deposit, the sperm bank refused because there was no law about who inherited sperm.[55]

If you mix I.V.F. and surrogate motherhood several more interesting possibilities arise:

- A woman with healthy ovaries but no uterus has her egg fertilized with her husband's sperm and then transferred to a surrogate mothers' womb (called "genuine surrogating").
- A woman with healthy uterus does not wish her egg to be fertilized, maybe because she has a genetic disease, buys an egg from a donor, has it fertilized with the husband's sperm and transfered to her uterus.
- A surrogate employed by a woman to be inseminated with her egg and her husband's sperm just to suit the egg donor's convenience. The woman wants a child, but doesn't want to be pregnant.
- A surrogate used to yield a desired genetic combination without any personal interaction—that is, by combining purchased egg and sperm, both from donors, and then transferring the embryo to the surrogate mother. The paying couple would sit back and wait for "their" baby to be born.

Think that's crazy? It gets crazier. With *embryo banking*, you could have the ultimate in family planning. You might decide to store your embryos early in your marriage for use at some later time. Anyone would do it, not just couples with a possible infertility problem. Embryo banking would rule out the added risk of genetic defect like Down's Syndrome which become more likely the later you have children.

With *embryo adoption*, you could either sell your extra embryos or buy them from others. Frozen embryos could be stockpiled. And the same would go for *egg* donations, as well as sperm donations. Buying embryos and using them in I.V.F. is *embryo transfer*. The use of donor embryos and donor eggs in I.V.F. is already a reality.[56] You could actually buy every component of a baby, maybe even sculpting its characteristics and temperament. Toffler's *Future Shock* vision of "babytoriums" where people pick the embryo of their choice is quickly on its way to being a vision come true.

Going back to Ramsey's fear of tampering with the genetic makeup of our children, there is actually a sperm bank called Repository for Germinal Choice that has advertised it has, on deposit, sperm from several Nobel Prize winners and other prominent, creative types. The ironic development of this organization has been its problem with screening the women inseminated. The mother of the first "Nobel Sperm Bank" baby was found to be a former convict who had lost custody of her children from a previous marriage due to her husband's abuse of them![57] This "Super-sperm" bank had taken so many pains with what type of person's sperm they would have and yet so few pains with what sort of person they inseminated. And because human nature is what it is, these surely are only a few of the inventive ways that will be found to take advantage of freezing these vital parts of procreation.

You can even mix A.I.D. and embryo transfer. It's already being done in America, some calling it *ovum transfer* and at least one clinic calling it "artificial embryonation." The situation would be one in which a childless couple would pay a fee to a woman who'd be inseminated with the husband's sperm. Then four or five days into the fertilization, the embryo would be flushed out and implanted in the wife. Ovum transfer could be an alternative to I.V.F. with an egg (ovum) donor. Its developers claim its success rates could reach fifty percent. Add that to the low cost and "nonsurgical" aspect of it, and ovum transfer might find its own niche in the world of biotechnical alternatives, if successful. Of course, ovum transfer would be a very different sort of A.I.D., one involving, not a male donor, but a female donor. The ethical questions, however, would be the same as for male A.I.D.

Other sci-fi sounding future possibilities include *cloning, egg fusion, fetal transfer,* and *genetic engineering* or *genetic splicing.*

Cloning is the possibility of replacing the nucleus of the egg with the nucleus of a body cell that contains the entire genetic code of the person it's taken from. The changed or "fertilized" egg would then be implanted in the womb, and in nine months you'd have an exact duplicate of the person the body cell was taken from.

Egg fusion would do away with any need for male input since the embryo would be created from two eggs, and would always produce a female. *Fetal transfer*, would be an actual "transfer" of a fetus from a woman who is contemplating abortion, for instance, to a woman who wants the child—"fetal adoption." Abortion, then, wouldn't have to result in the death of a fetus but merely a transfer to another womb—mechanical or human. And *genetic marking* or *splicing* would allow us to have "quality control" over the way our kids turned out. . . . These techniques are more than just strange impossible ideas. Researchers, using animals, are now experimenting with all these possibilities.[58]

The list could go on. There seems to be no end to the variations that can be attempted with the I.V.F. technology; the question for researchers seems to be only, "What might work?"

If *genetic engineering* is part of the techniques escaping from I.V.F.'s Pandora's box, then *genetic abortion* will become an issue. Soon, we very possibly will be able to screen young embryos for hereditary diseases. We can already screen the fetus with the *amniocentesis* test, which is used to detect severe chromosome disorders like Down's Syndrome. (The option of therapeutic abortion is usually offered in tandem with the test if such a case is found . . . another agonizing choice our new technology offers us.) And a *fetoscopy*, done with fiber-optic cameras, sophisticated measuring instruments and ultrasound, can potentially be used to detect other hereditary diseases like sickle-cell anemia and hemophilia.[59]

Do we or do we not abort embryos so afflicted? As in the

abortion issue, genetic abortion will bring us face to face with the how we view life, and how we see the status of the embryo. The best answer, of course, would be to cure the embryo—which is potentially the future answer. The fetoscopy, already used to give blood transfusions to diseased fetuses, has the potential for introducing medicines, or even healthy genetic materials into the womb in order to treat genetic diseases. Right now skeletal defects and cosmetic defects like cleft palates can be seen in the womb.[60] But as long as we cannot cure these embryos with genetic diseases such as Tay-Sachs syndrome, Down's Syndrome, or other physical and mental handicaps, abortion will be offered as a curious form of "cure"—not for making the patient better, but for bringing the patient's existence to the end. Some will argue about quality of life, quantity of suffering. Some will argue that we can alleviate some diseases altogether in this matter, and some believe that the parent's welfare is of first concern. As infertile couples, we shudder at the idea of ending life, even though we cannot help but worry about deformities. A call must be made to work toward curing those genetic malformations with *real* cures.

The I.V.F. implications for the family may be even more complex than those of A.I.D. With in vitro, surrogating, embryo transfer, embryo freezing, and artificial insemination, it is actually possible for a child to have as many as five "parents": the egg donor, the sperm donor, the surrogate who bears the child, and the couple who raises it.

One quote shows the craziness of the complications in all its cosmic absurdity. In his book *Utopian Motherhood*, Dr. Robert Francoer poses this problem:

> A barren woman, citizen of Russia, receives an ovarian transplant from a black citizen of Nigeria. Married to a sterile . . . native of the Australian bush country, she is artificially inseminated with frozen semen from an Eskimo . . . but the Russian woman has difficulty carrying the child, so she arranges for an American Indian woman to serves as a substitute mother. Puzzle out, if you

will—if you can, the racial and national constitution of the off-spring, its citizenship, and its two (?) parents.[61]

SURROGATE MOTHERHOOD

What about surrogating? This may be the most visible of all today's applications of I.V.F. technology. And that only adds to its controversial nature. We are already hearing and reading about it—surrogating is part of our TV dramas and our newspaper headlines. And the ethical questions abound. Is the surrogate an "incubator-for-hire?" Is she "selling" her body? Is she selling her baby? Is what she's doing legal? What if she changes her mind and wants to keep the baby? And who takes final responsibility for the child if something goes wrong?

First, how should the surrogate woman view herself? If she took an emotionally detached view—if that were possible—how could that affect the baby? (At least one psychologist, a Canadian, opposes surrogating because he believes the fetus is sensitive to the emotions of the mother—and the needed "distancing" a surrogate mother must do from the baby within her might cause psychological problems for the baby.)[62] How could she see herself as anything but a "mother?"

Second, how would the "adoptive" couple view the surrogate? According to Dr. Janet McDowell, a British religious ethicist, the couple would have only two choices of how to treat the surrogate—viewing her as a means to their reproductive end or creating a new form of extended family. Dr. McDowell believes it would be difficult to structure a surrogate situation in such a way that the surrogate would be fully respected as a person. But her biggest argument revolves around whether we want to "encourage women to perceive procreative capacities as mere services for hire."[63]

What about the legal issues? Is the woman selling her baby? Most states have laws prohibiting such trading, bartering or buying and selling infant children. There is always the problem of coercion, the women promised the necessities of life in return for the surrender of the child.[64] That would be one of the many abuses surrogating is open to. Yet the law doesn't clearly grapple with any of the surrogate situations. And it must.

As syndicated columnist Ellen Goodman summed it up, foremost among arguments against surrogating is the ethical question raised . . . "that surrogating is a business that encourages people to regard parents as customers rather than caretakers . . . motherhood as biological work on a reproduction line. . . ."[65]

And then, there is the question no one wants to think about. What if the baby is deformed? What if nobody wants it?

It's already happened. And stranger yet, one case was resolved on a TV talk show, the Phil Donahue Show, in 1983, in full soap opera dimensions. A New York man paid a married woman from Detroit ten thousand dollars to be inseminated with his sperm, bear the resulting child, and give him custody. But the baby was born with a severe infection and with defects that suggested retardation. Neither of the parties wanted the child. To make matters worse, the man refused to authorize the hospital to treat the baby's medical condition. According to the New York Times, the hospital went to court and won permission to care for the baby.

Meanwhile . . . the surrogate mother and her husband demanded their money. The New York man insisted on blood and tissue tests to prove his paternity before he would pay. He announced on the Phil Donahue Show that the tests proved the child was not his. And at that point the surrogate mother and husband—and apparent real father—decided to keep the child.[66]

But what if they hadn't? The verdict is still out on what will happen with our "mistakes."

SEX SELECTION

And then, how about choosing your baby's sex? Would you do it if you could? Most of us would consider it, figuring the decision wouldn't affect anyone but our direct family. It is already an experimental option, as science is learning how to separate the X and Y chromosomes. One California research company, claiming a seventy-five percent success rate selecting male babies, has actually patented its procedure, forcing clinics to buy licenses from it in order to offer the "service."[67]

But would choosing the sex of our children be smart? At one Dallas clinic that offers this option, over two-thirds of the couples requests boys.[68] Made-to-order firstborn sons? That idea has many feminists, religious leaders, and doctors concerned. Population-wise and sociological-wise, such an imbalance would be catastrophic, bordering on just plain dumb. Of course, some researchers disagree saying that such a situation would never take place. Wyoming reproductive physiologist Ronald Ericsson states that less than one percent of the six thousand parents who've contacted him wanted to preselect their firstborn. He says, "Most were parents who already had two children of the same sex, and wanted only one more child—of the opposite sex . . . American couples want small families and they want one child of each sex. There's no more to it than that."[69] Yet, concern is still real and widespread. Two Japanese professors, for instance, who've developed a technique which they say assures the birth of females are so concerned with the technique's inherent problems that they've asked the medical ethics committee of their university to pass on the ethical issues involved with their accomplishment.[70]

Intricate, ambiguous, explosive, perplexing, unmanageable . . . unsolvable. All these adjectives describe how the ethical issues of the new biotechnology can look to anybody who tackles it. And when all the techniques hold personal implications, well, those adjectives multiply.

Maybe you won't be able to decide your personal ethical issue easily. Maybe it hits too close to home. These kinds of issues are the ones we'd love to have someone else decide for us. But no one else can. I don't presume—and can't—to tell you what judgments to make. Some seem obvious, others quite ambiguous. But it doesn't seem fair that we have to be thrown into an ethical dilemma in the middle of our medical one. Of course, fairness doesn't seem to have anything to do with this whole crisis, does it?

One thing holds true, though—past our personal choices. We *must* be aware of all that is going on around us. And then we must add that to what is going on within us. Then whatever our answers, whatever our decisions, I do believe we must take a vocal part toward shaping more ethical and legal boundaries for the new procedures, now that we know about the explosion in biotechnology and the potential power that much of the new knowledge will give people over society. Because of all we've gone through, we are more informed than most of society outside the medical world. Whether we decide against these new procedures, whether we like some and worry about others, whether we find the new possibilities exciting and worthwhile, we'll have an opinion. Alvin Toffler was right when he said, "Despite profound ethical questions about whether we should, the fact remains that scientific curiosity is, itself, one of the most powerful driving forces in our society."[71] So, responsibility is the key word—in a personal way and in a cultural way. Especially since there's no putting any of these amazing possibilities back into that Pandora's Box.

Chapel, *the white sign says on the door. I stop, gaze numbly at it. The neatly hand-painted sign looks so out of place in the modern hall of the hospital. I stand staring at it for a moment, then stumble in.*

The place is dark and I fumble for a light switch. Instantly, the room is bathed in muted light and stained glass reflections. And I slide into a pew.

The atmosphere is familiar, warm, tranquil.

Yet there's nothing tranquil about me. My best friend had just had a miscarriage. The pregnancy had been miraculous, everyone had said. And now she had lost the baby. But she's fine the doctor said. Just fine.

I sit staring at the stained glass figures surrounding me, their robes, beards, sandals. And I know I'm not fine at all.

I close my eyes a moment, and breathe deeply. She had waited forever to tell me about being pregnant, worried how I'd respond. Wonderful, I had said and only half meant it. Hating myself for selfish thoughts. Denying to myself, to her, to God, how sad her happiness had made me.

And now. Oh now. How could I have felt that way? What am I turning into? This infertility is a nightmare. It's not fair. Nothing's fair. I was angry then. I'm angry now. And I just can't deny it anymore. Not here, not in such a place.

It's not fair, Lord. Do you hear?!

The silence is deafening. I'm alone with all the stained glass people. Out of the corner of my eye, I recognize Abraham, and I remember the story of how God "blessed" him and his "barren" wife Sarah with a son in their old age. Barren . . . "blessed with children" . . . "cursed with barrenness." I wince.

Why, God? *I find myself praying.* I feel so awful, so angry! So ashamed. Nothing makes sense. Life doesn't. You don't. Nothing. *Leaning back against the pew's cold wood, I look up.*

What is happening? Why are we having to go through this? Have I done something wrong?

Are you not "blessing" us for some reason?

Why do I feel my prayers are going absolutely nowhere? You are so silent, so far away. . . .

"What are we supposed to believe, God?" I ask aloud. "How are we supposed to feel? What are we supposed to DO?" It seems I used to know, *I frown, looking down vacantly at my hands clenched together in my lap.* Faith used to be a simple thing. But now, I'm so confused. And so disappointed. And so . . . different than I used to be. *I sigh. "Everything's so different," I murmur. And I don't know what to do with how I feel. I want to believe God's in control . . . but if You are . . . I think, looking back up, and if You love me. . . .*

"Please, God, I just want to understand . . . I just want . . ." I feel my eyes well up with tears and I fight it, taking a long, slow breath. The chapel seems darker somehow, the air filled with my questions. And all I'm filled with is a great, hollow sadness.

Here, even here, infertility has taken over. Tell me, Lord, how did this happen? And where did You go?

I look up at the stained glass panel above the altar. A young Mary, cradling baby Jesus. The angels are hovering and singing. I try like crazy to feel something, to hear something. To know something for sure. Yet, instead, I wonder if I'll keep asking questions forever . . . or worse, if I'll give up and stop asking at all.

HOW WILL THIS AFFECT MY FAITH?

The Spiritual Crisis—*A Personal View*

It's one thing to talk about how infertility affects such things as emotions, social pressures, ethics, and trips to the hospital. It's quite another to talk about how it affects my spiritual life.

Why? Fear. Fear that my faith was in danger. To examine something so deeply a part of me and realize that it might not be working just right is scary. To even admit being angry at God is hard.

So I denied that I was. But the little questions kept seeping in. . . . We didn't do anything to make this happen so who, then, is to blame? Why is this happening? And where do I direct this awful anger?

No answers.

So the anger directed itself. I've gone through bouts of depression that made my insides numb. I've picked fights with my husband. I've stared confused and disappointed at the sky and wondered what was happening, this great, awful silence filling the empty space around me—and in me. Where was God? Where was justice and fairness? I just couldn't make myself take the next step of pulling out my faith and examining it against this crisis I was going through.

You see, I was worried it wouldn't hold up. Some people have the gift of faith, never questioning through the trenches. Some don't worry about faith at all, strolling through life with a shrug and a roll of the dice. I am neither of those. For the longest time, questioning God seemed wrong. Surely my faith wasn't very healthy if it couldn't weather a life crisis without a bunch of questions and emotional harangues. And the "answers" I had heard hadn't helped much:

"It must be God's will."

"You know, maybe you're being punished for something."

"Maybe it's all just fate. Maybe there isn't any God out there."

"You just have to have enough faith. That's all."

The unfaced questions are bad enough, forcing us into our own little pockets of personal hell, but most of the answers we hear only fan the fire. And as I listened, I wondered if my faith was going to hold up under the strain.

And I know I'm not alone. What is it about infertility, anyway? Can't it stay out of at least one area of our lives? Why can't this one area remain untouched, a source of help instead of hurt?

Yet once more, as with all the other issues of infertility we've covered, I'm reminded that our crisis is an unusual one—a different one, because the whole infertility crisis has been one without definition, without framework or past experience to point to. The only thing we can be sure of is that it *will* seep into every space of our lives. And as it trickles into our spiritual space, a spotlight is thrown on the big questions of life itself. And the faith that probably would be a source of comfort in other crises becomes part of the crisis itself—forcing us to take another look at the very bottom line of belief. As Dr. Lewis Smedes has put it so well:

. . . [E]very infertile woman who has prayed for conception while she took painful note of irresponsible girls awaiting unwanted babies has felt that she must wait on the incomprehensible pleasure of a whimsical Creator.[1]

The incomprehensible pleasure of a whimsical God? It can sure seem that way. One couple after years of trying gives birth. And with a shake of their heads and a prayer of thanks, they put the spiritual question to rest. Another couple gets the news they will never be able to have children of their own and are forced to let the dream die. They don't understand, but if faith teaches us anything, it teaches us to deal with death, in whatever form.

Another couple finally gives birth and the baby dies. Another miscarries again and again. And still another must keep facing a long line of decisions and testing and treatments that get more complicated by the month. In another time, such couples would finally hit a brick wall in their infertility treatment and sum it up to fate, to God, to life. But now technology has, in many cases, handed such couples the chord to their dreams and left it up to them when to pull the plug. And then the question becomes harder: When, in the midst of why?

God. Incomprehensible? Whimsical? Inscrutable? Mysterious? Unpredictable? What happened to Loving? Just? Personal? The *new* adjectives are beginning to make more sense than the old ones.

These are the thoughts I could not make myself face honestly. The world should make sense. My life should make sense. My faith should make sense! Yet I was beginning to believe that nothing made sense.

Lewis Smedes knows what I mean. He knows about the incomprehensible. In this book *Forgive and Forget*, under a chapter entitled "Forgiving God," he tells of his own infertility experience that forced him to face his questions about God head-on. After going to fertility clinics here and abroad, he and his wife, Doris, had gone through years of waiting with no answers: "We made love whenever the thermometer told us the time was at hand. We played our parts in the unromantic comedy of artificial insemination. We prayed in between." And then she finally became pregnant. What they had wanted most they were getting. It seemed that their prayers were answered.

But in her seventh month, labor began. The doctor told them the baby would be badly deformed and to prepare themselves. Then miraculously, the baby was normal. Another prayer seemed to be answered. Yet before Lewis and Doris had time to savor the joy, they got the news. The baby wasn't breathing well. In a very short time, they were burying their child. And the irony and the hurt and the questions set in:

> Why, after the night of getting ready to love a deformed child; why after the surprise that even doctors called a miracle; why, miracle done, was death the punch line? I felt as if I were the butt of a cruel divine joke. Would I end up hating God?[2]

Hating God? Maybe we all do. On the sly. From time to time. But if it's true, and I do hate God at times, I think it must be the way I'd hate a trusted friend—as if my most important friend had become my worst enemy. Could that be? Like a close friend who has done you wrong, you wouldn't know where to put your anger. You'd be confused because this friend has meant so much to you, has vowed to be there, to reach out to you, but now seems to be standing passively by when you need him the most. How else can you feel about that friend? Your feelings would be a crazy mixture of hate, of disappointment, of anger, of confusion—but also, I think, of a hurt love in search of reconciliation.

Most of us feel this way, however we may look at the spiritual side of life. There are certain things we expect out of our faith, and among those is that it should be a source of security, of strength and comfort—of answers. And when we seem to see evidence that it isn't, all of life is suddenly covered with question marks. Only the most honest and brave will begin to confront the questions, as this woman did in a letter to the editor of the RESOLVE newsletter:

> . . . I can only see [my infertility] as some sort of punishment from God, and I don't have any idea for what I am being pun-

ished . . . People tell me that perhaps God is answering my prayers, then why should one bother to pray in the first place? People portray an image of God who can supervise the world, but because of "free-will" or whatever, cannot intervene. If so, what good is God? Why should we pay any attention to a God who has no power? . . . [W]hy doesn't he help me? I cannot see my infertility as a part of any great plan for good, and it has driven a wedge between me and my God. . . .[3]

These are the important issues. These are the ones that stare back at us as we sit in the dark. Why isn't life clear? What is God doing? And why?

An innate part of us rushes to God's defense just as another part of us is railing against him. And some of us feel a need to take such defense to an extreme. In his book *When Bad Things Happen to Good People*, Rabbi Harold S. Kushner speaks of forgiving God, but only in the sense that we cannot blame God for everything. He believes that some things are even too hard for God. Such a God worries about us, is up there cheering us on like a well-meaning grandfather, but ultimately he really can't do much. Rabbi Kushner places the issue of God's whole character in an either/or sentence. Judging from all the hurt and pain in the world, Rabbi Kushner believes he is forced to choose between a good God who is not all-powerful and an all-powerful God who is not good. So he chooses one who isn't all-powerful.

Such a God, though, would be a weak one, and forgiving him would be easy. Yet such a God doesn't seem to be much of a "God." Strong, just, wise, *all-powerful*—these words are integral to our very basic, innate definition of "God."

But allowing God to be totally God-like is risky. And that's why it's easy to picture him otherwise, if it gets him—and us— off the hook. Because if we venture that he is all-powerful, then we must take the next step and ask, if he's all-powerful, why doesn't he make everything all right? And that takes guts. Reducing God to an "either/or" is safe. Most people would rather not face such questions for fear of the answers.

And that's why I've put off facing them for so long. I wanted to protect my faith, not examine it. I was afraid that if I couldn't reduce it to an easy either/or, that if I couldn't be satisfied with its loose ends, I might lose my faith.

But as I've been forced to contemplate it all, I realize that I've been propping up my present faith with toothpicks, and then standing guard over it for fear of it toppling over. What kind of belief is that? At best a weak, powerless, defensive one.

Okay. So. I've talked myself into facing my questions. I'm going to let myself openly doubt—and "doubting," in this context, must mean to honestly examine—risk or no risk.

Oh, I know the "right" answers. A lifetime of church-going can offer lots of advisers and lots of fodder for quick-fix solutions. But as I've begun to face my feelings and my questions, I realize how very personal the questions and the answers are, and, ultimately, how I—in my own personal way—must address them. Alone. So I made my own list, and, not surprisingly, the questions are very close to the ones the letter-writer earlier posed:

Why me? Do I deserve this?

Is God a loving God? If so, why doesn't he help?

Are we supposed to learn something specific from this?

Why pray if it doesn't seem to help?

What *about* healing and miracles and such? And all the answers people offer? Are they right when they tell me it's just a matter of faith?

What is life about if not to bear and raise a family?

Slowly, I began to examine these questions, in search of the answers that were right for me . . . honestly examining them in the midst of my doubt, my anger, and my fear. And I was surprised at what I found.

Why me? Do I deserve this?

Job is one of our culture's all-time examples of world-class, undeserved suffering. If there ever was a man who didn't "deserve" to have trouble, it was Job. Yet Job got trouble with both barrels as he lost his children, his farm, his livestock, and his health. All he had left was a deadly practical wife who advised him to curse God and die. None of it, though, made sense, because Job knew he had done nothing wrong, nothing to deserve any of what had happened.

Then his friends came to see him. They felt, as most of us do, that they must offer some sort of solution to this crisis. Logic dictated, they decided that Job must have brought all this on himself. Yet Job knew his own heart well enough to know he hadn't. He began to notice slowly that evil and good aren't always punished and rewarded in this life. And yet this unjustly wronged man held on, believing beyond all reason and logic.

Did we do something to deserve these years of infertility? Over and over, people like Job's friends set up this idea: If you are prospering, you are being rewarded for your goodness. But if a plague of locusts descends on you or a brick wall falls on you as you innocently stroll by—or if you find yourselves infertile—*you* caused it through your badness.

It's a convenient theory, one that makes life quite simple. The only problem is it's not true. "Bad" people are consistently prospering all around us and have done so throughout history. And still we cling to this idea. What if Job's friends were right? What if we are rewarded for being good and having faith and punished when we are bad and don't have faith? Who in their right mind would choose anything else but faith? We'd be conditioned to seek God, like trained monkeys—not through having the freedom to choose between two attractive alternatives, but through knowing by instinct what would keep us living the "good life."

Such a system *would* "work," in a sense . . . most of us would be believers. The question, though, would be: *Why* would we be believers? Because we wanted to know God? Or because we wanted what we wanted? The answer is as obvious as the choice. And so is the flaw in the whole idea.

I don't deserve what has happened. But I don't deserve for

it not to happen. And I think realizing that is a big step. One that still tastes a little sour in my mouth. Obviously, our goodness and faith are *not* redeemable for the "good life." They don't seem to help at all. So—why choose to believe? Why *should* I believe in a God who has such a strange way of showing his love?

Right now, I can't get these questions off my mind. Maybe it's because we are at the point in our infertility where we are contemplating giving up treatment. And inexplicably intertwined with that decision is the somewhat irrational fear that when I give up on medicine, I will also give up the idea that God cares about what happens to me, that he loves me. It scares me to death to question that. If I open up this idea for examination, will I begin to believe he doesn't love me? And how could I keep believing if I don't believe he loves me?

I must not be the first to wonder about his love. What do people do with these feelings? I can stand questioning most anything, but this. Just like Job, I've called out over and over for an explanation, just enough to understand, to get me through. . . . But when Job waited for an answer, God sidestepped the question. God instead reminded Job of his power, his majesty, his creation—who *he* was. What did God *want* from Job?

What do *we* want from God? Famed Oxford scholar and writer C. S. Lewis once wrote:

> We want not so much a father in heaven, as a grandfather in heaven—whose plan for the universe was such that it might be said at the end of the day, "A good time was had by all."
>
> I should very much like to live in a universe which was governed on such lines, but since it is abundantly clear that I don't, and since I have reason to believe nevertheless that God is love, I conclude that my conception of love needs correction. . . .[4]

Well, maybe that's what I need—my conception of love corrected. And maybe even my conception of God. Could the message be that love is part of what has been happening to us?

And could it be that if my faith can stretch enough to cover that message that I'll learn a lesson in such love . . .? It's a tall order. I can already see, though, that I have a lot to learn about love from God's standpoint. And a lot to learn about God.

Are we supposed to learn something specific from this?

Well, since the infertility is a very definite part of our lives, could our suffering, then, be to teach us something specific? I know the usual qualities that adversity can give a person: perseverance, patience, compassion, insight, wisdom—*character.* Right now, my head is agreeing, but my heart is having nothing to do with the idea.

Character. Reminds me of my long-ago teenage response after losing a race for high school cheerleader. My mother wisely pointed out that the experience was good for my character—to which I replied that I had enough character, thank you very much—I'd rather be cheerleader.

Are we talking character? I'd rather have a baby, my heart responds. If this infertility experience is to teach me something, it better be good.

Obviously, I have a hard time seeing some sort of "greater good" coming from the ordeal of infertility and even less from the possibility of my never having children. The real question seems to be whether I believe that God could make a situation in which any hurt, no matter how big or extended, could be worth it. Dr. Bruce Shelley poses the question this way:

> Let us suppose that God's resources are so much beyond what we can imagine that he can produce a situation in which anything was understandable. The problem of evil, then, is the problem of faith. Do we believe in a God big enough to make any suffering seem worthwhile?[5]

Can my faith stretch far enough to take in such an idea? I believe so, even if it seems mostly an intellectual exercise. As before, my heart wants to *know* the greater good in order to decide for itself. But Dr. Shelley is saying that faith is *not* knowing, yet believing anyway. And that's one mighty hard idea to grasp and hold on to when you're hurting.

C. S. Lewis once called pain, "God's megaphone." He believed that pain and suffering shouts—that it's a message from God, all right, but it's a general one that makes us ponder what is really going on in the world. Do we think that the purpose of living is to have a good time, to live happily ever after? Is that what life is for? As C. S. Lewis would probably reply, if you think so, you'd have to do so with your fingers in your ears to drown out the bellow of the megaphone.

So suffering is to get our attention? It certainly does that. But to what end? As Philip Yancey explains in his book, *Where Is God When It Hurts,* suffering takes us a step further than just getting our attention. It will almost undoubtedly force us to make a choice. As he puts it, ". . . I can hate God for allowing such misery. Or, on the other hand, it can drive me to Him."[6]

More than not, we find ourselves in a never-never land buffeted between these two extremes—mad one moment, reaching out the next. But even those of us who are ultimately pulled toward God want desperately to believe that there is some specific message, some cause for our suffering, so we can do something about it and get rid of it *now.* What did I do? Just tell me, and I'll do whatever it takes to make it right. . . . But that doesn't seem to be how it all works. Yancey tells of being with suffering people who react much like this:

> [They] torment themselves with the question, "What is God trying to teach me?" Or, they may writhe, "How can I muster up enough faith to get rid of this illness. How can I get God to rescue me?" Maybe they have it all wrong. Maybe God isn't trying to tell us anything specific each time we hurt . . . The message may simply be that we live in a world with fixed laws, like everyone else.[7]

"In a world of fixed laws." What would that mean for us? One idea I'm consistently confronted with is the idea that God decides who gets a child and who doesn't—the idea of a child as a "blessing" only given to those God chooses. It's a somewhat subconscious thought that is alive and well in the minds of many believers, one that makes us wonder about punishment and favoritism and guilt. As psychologist Dr. James Dobson plainly puts the problem: "If a child is evidence of God's approval, then is the absence of a child evidence of God's disapproval? I think not. And yet there are many women who draw that assumption."[8] And it is a very easy assumption to draw. I often find myself asking: *Could* this infertility be what God wants for us? In all honesty, I can't say that it isn't. The will of God defies explanation, it seems. But if I do not believe that, over all, God is sending specific signals with suffering, I wouldn't believe that this suffering—our infertility—was specifically pointed at us. Instead, I believe we're living in a world of fixed laws—and one of those laws is the natural law of procreation.

In her little book *Beyond Heartache*, Mari Haynes explains her belief that God doesn't have control of the reins of everyone's specific pregnancy. Procreation, she states, is as integral a part of nature's laws as any you can name, and therefore should be viewed as other natural laws:

> . . . [A] young, unmarried girl who becomes pregnant has not been "zapped" with a pregnancy from God. Instead, she has used the prerogative God gave her to begin a new life. Neither is God punishing you by keeping you from getting pregnant; something is interfering with the natural law of conception.[9]

God has set the laws of nature in motion. Why would he break the normal laws of nature on a regular basis on this one law and not on any other? And although I must believe he *can* do it, just as I believe he can break *any* of nature's laws, I do not believe he does it as a rule. Maybe this is the sort of answer we hear from people who *must* have answers, who feel they should be able to explain the inexplicable. But that just may not be humanly possible at times.

Still, many people feel a very natural pull to believe that everything that happens to us is from God. It seems, though, that it actually might be dangerous to try to find comfort in an overly-simplistic acceptance of our infertility being God's doing.

Why? Well, the danger of such an outlook is the danger of looking at all pain and suffering in the world as being straight from God. We'd resign ourselves to a form of fatalism. Sit back and let the diseases kill us off, stay put when a hurricane is coming our way. Instead, it seems that we are called to battle the awful things that confront us. And in that vein, we are certainly right to battle the problems of infertility.

What about healing and miracles and such? What about the answers people offer? Are they right when they say it is just a matter of enough faith?

Some of the confusing, most frustrating experiences of our infertility crisis are the comments we field from the people around us. They tell us of their cousin Myrtle and her miraculous conception, or they give "spiritual" advice concerning our situation. I sometimes think that such statements as *"You'd be able to have a baby if you just had enough faith"* and *"Maybe you're being punished"* is our way of battling the unknowable. We by nature must understand, must have control. And we are scared stiff by the idea that there is mystery in our lives— that God is just as he claims to be, supernatural in the best sense of the word. Yet, bound as we are in our natural laws, we feel helpless. And so, again, if we can't have control of a situation, we try to explain it away.

But we all know stories of couples who have had miraculous things happen to them as they've coped with infertility. And we can't help wondering if there is that *something* we might do to make it happen for us. *How do we understand the role that we as believers play in the miraculous? Can we make such things happen if we have enough faith? Does God pick "favorites" he decides to help?* I see a lot of truth in the way Yancey probed these questions:

> . . . We seem to reserve our shiniest merit badges for those who
> have been healed . . . with the frequent side-effect of causing un-
> healed ones to feel as though God has passed them by. We make
> faith not an attitude of trust in something unseen but a route to
> get something *seen*—something magical and stupendous, like a
> miracle. . . . Faith includes the supernatural, but it also includes
> daily, dependent trust in spite of results . . . a belief without solid
> proof. God is not mere magic . . .[10]

Miracles, however they happen and whoever they happen
to, are exceptions, not rules. That's the nature of miracles. To
make them something we can earn with the right poundage of
faith is to belittle the wondrous, to have control over the supernatural. And in effect, if we were able to do this, if we could
make miracles the rule, we'd have to redefine what a miracle
is, because it wouldn't be a "miracle" anymore. Either that or
redefine who *we* are, since we could control miracles. . . .

Job's friends would fit right in here. And none of us are much
different. We all want a prepackaged set of spiritual rules to
live by. Life would be a lot easier if we knew exactly what was
needed to make things the way we want them to be. To sum
up someone's suffering with statements like "You must have
done something wrong" is an attempt to control life, to have
simple answers to difficult questions. It's safe. It's putting the
Creator of the universe in our hip pocket, an attempt to fill the
unquenchable need we have to explain the universe to each
other.

In essence, we cannot allow for mystery. Especially if it is
painful mystery. It's easier to let someone else sum up our
problem for us than to confront it and examine it through our
own eyes.

But if we allow for mystery, can we still confront the situation
and examine it? I think so. Because there's a difference between
explaining and explaining away. I really believe the truth in
Malcolm Muggeridge's thought, "To believe greatly, it is necessary to doubt greatly," and I'm convinced that such honest
searching may mean the difference between mere suffering and

suffering that causes deeper faith. Acceptance of the mystery may *be* part and parcel of the answer that comes, but it will be much more satisfying if it comes as a result of personal thought.

So how do we weather those "right" answers and decide for ourselves how such ideas fit into our own crisis?

The first rule is not to play it safe. Not to put God in a handy-sized box, and not to expect easy answers to hard questions. And then maybe the second rule is to be open to answers you aren't expecting. And the third? Very possibly, not to listen to your own set of "Job's friends" no matter how sincere they are, and instead, to examine each idea against your own feelings and beliefs.

Why pray if it doesn't seem to help?

When my husband and I began our infertility quest, I prayed about our situation a lot. But very soon, I noticed it became a pleading, a monologue that exhausted me, physically and spiritually. So I stopped praying about it.

That may sound like I've given up on prayer. On the contrary. What has happened is that I've learned more about prayer. What *is* prayer for? As I began looking at that question through different eyes, I began considering prayer on a deeper, different level. Could prayer be more of a time when we are just being with God? Could it be a time for getting in touch with our spiritual sides as we reach out to God? It's got to be more than a way to remind an absent-minded God what we need, or else we reduce prayer to the same get-what-we-want sort of mentality that misses the whole meaning of prayer and faith and spirituality.

And this may be where we began. When we were discussing Job, I asked the question, *why believe?* If believing is not going to get us any favors, if it's not going to keep us any safer than Job, then why would anyone believe? There *has* to be more.

Dr. Paul Brand, a doctor well-known for his work with pain, was asked to think of some believers who had gone through extreme suffering. Had their suffering caused a deeper faith or ruined the faith they had? Dr. Brand explained that those who dwelt on "cause," hung up on questions such as the ones we know intimately—who to blame, why is this happening?— these people became bitter and drifted away from their faith into despair. But those who shifted into "response," who had gotten past the "why?" and had moved into "How will I respond to this awful thing?"—those found themselves believing more deeply than ever before.[11]

And maybe this is where the chapter turns. Do I question the *cause* or do I begin working on the *response?* Do I focus on why this is happening or how my faith helps me cope? The natural reaction to any crisis is to search for the cause of the pain before deciding how to respond. But in concentrating on "cause," will I end up embittered? And if I ultimately find no concrete, simple answers, will I be comforted by my embitterment? It seems I must make a leap if I am to keep believing, but the chasm is wide and so full of half-answered questions.

I think my choice may ultimately hinge on a brutally honest look at *why I am believing.* Like praying, is it to get what I want or to get to know God? Very few of us are ever made to search ourselves so honestly for an answer to that one. Yet, it may mean the difference between staying stuck in "cause," or being able to move on to "response" and spiritual health.

It's so hard to get away from the why of the crisis. And even after the in-depth look at my questions, I am still tugged both ways. At times my anger and my dreams won't let go even now. But I want to believe that the world is a place where innocents are hurt not by God but because of wrong choices, imperfect bodies, and a tumbledown world—not because God is powerless, but because he must give us room to choose freely. I can't believe that God stayed up one night and decided that we'd never have a child of our own. Instead, I believe that the laws of nature were set in motion and very, very rarely have they ever been preempted, and I am not presumptuous enough to demand such attention. I must believe, though, we *could* be healed of our physical imperfections, but I cannot expect it or demand it. And I will not demand such attention before I believe. That, I'm convinced, is faith.

So, *cause or response?* One fear keeps pounding in my mind, as I ponder the choice. What will happen if I stay stuck on cause? Will the end result be that embitterment? The crisis has the estimate power to either push me toward God or away from him, it seems. I must make a choice. If I keep pushing the "why?" if I keep blaming God, then I may end up a double-loser. I may never have a child, and I will be alone, separated from him. I will allow one disappointment to shatter my faith, to keep me from the one relationship that lasts—past motherhood, past marriage, past it all. There is a pain that is worse than having a friend's two-year-old bound happily into your lap. It's the pain of not feeling anyone there when friends and child and everyone has left. For Job, the answer was not an answer, it was a *presence*. If I go the way of embitterment, however valid my reasons seem to be, I'll be alone. An alone that is pain in itself. I already know that terrible aloneness of railing against God, the gnawing bitterness of feeling mad and searching for someone to blame. But, as one struggler has put it so eloquently, my "arms are too short to box with God." They weren't meant for boxing with him, and my swings are only tiring out my soul. Such a feeling for only a short time is awful. As a way of life it is intolerable. It's not what I'm made for, and not what I want.

So even as I still hurt, and even as I look back, still straining over the leap, I choose to believe anyway. I choose response. What does it take to get to this point? For Rabbi Kushner and the Smedes, through their individual struggles, it was a form of forgiving God—for our sake, not his, for what we do not understand in light of what we feel about his presence. For me, it has been a process of thinking until I couldn't think anymore, of feeling until I couldn't feel anymore—until I was able to think and feel on a different level altogether.

A great deal of mystery remains. I can talk all day about how

God works with us and how we respond, but obviously, I can only talk of what makes sense to me through the light of my own knowledge of God. That must be the way God wants it. We can see such an idea in the way he answered Job. Yet even through such a seeming "non-answer," we can also see that God cared for Job. What God asked of Job was his faith, his trust.

In our anger, there is no way we think we can do that. Ours is usually a conditional trust at best, hinging on the outcome. We forget that this Supreme Being we believe in and the whole conception of him is described with the word "supernatural." We demand the logical, the answerable. But the true essence of faith is that things are not logical, that there is a reality that cannot be seen. Great mystery. We forget that. We won't let God or this life be a mystery, and I've decided that I must.

Is there a possibility that all of this isn't true? If I understand correctly, that's part of faith, too. There's no way to prove a matter of faith, really. It's an innate truth you either grasp with both hands or let slip away. It's all in the believing anyway. A way to say it's all right—when your head is screaming that everything is all wrong, and yet an echo deep in your heart is whispering that, somehow, it can still be okay.

Past it all, past the doubts, the theories, the seeming illogic of the choice, I keep going back to the simple ideas that will not let me go:

There is a Creator.

He loves me, and wants to know me.

He cares enough to give me freedom.

Suffering makes no sense except in the way it reminds us of life's true reality.

Faith isn't made of logic and sense, but of believing any-how, of leaping into the dark.

I have a choice whether I want to believe.

Life is for more than having babies.

I am living for a reason.

I need to love God back.

Evelyn Underhill, a famous English writer, believed we spend most of our lives conjugating three verbs: *to Want*, *to Have*, and *to Do*. Yet:

> None of these verbs have any ultimate significance, except so far as they are transcended by and included in, the fundamental verb, to "Be." And that Being, not wanting, having, doing, is the essence of spiritual life.[12]

I *want* a child. It is one of many dreams I *have*. And I will *do* almost anything it takes to have our own. But most of all—now—I will *be*. The infertility crisis is one that can easily get us all tied up with having and wanting and doing. We forget that *being* is the important thing. Who we are is what matters.

So add another to the list of simple truths:

My being is important to the Supreme Being. The Great "I Am" cares that I am—above all that I have, want or do.

And that's something. Maybe everything.

My faith has already changed, though not changed enough, for the most part yet, I suppose. I still feel wounded, and probably will for as long as we are still grappling with infertility and its impact on our future. But now I have the hope that the wounds might heal back stronger than before. Choosing to stay open to my faith doesn't mean I do not still want a child, or that I give up. And it doesn't mean I'll not have relapses into my own little personal hells of peer pressure, of self-pity, of slamming doors and shaking fists. But if this works out the way I think it will work out, I'll be relapsing less and less, and finding my faith more and more—on the same level that Job did. Not finding answers, so much as "presence." And if so, I'll remember that this isn't all there is, that life isn't for having, doing, and wanting. And on the days that I do, I'll find that God is God, and that he loves me—Being to being. And I'll find that such belief is sufficient. For the moment. For the day. For the future, children or no.

"You're here!" my sister smiles as she hugs me and ushers me through her front door. "How long has it been? Way too long, right, Benjamin?" I look down at her three-year-old who is clinging and grinning and nodding. "How long did it take you to get here? Have a nice trip?" she goes on, as Benjamin scampers away.

"About four hours. And yes, it was nice and quiet and I really enjoyed just cruising along," I answer as we walk into the kitchen and dining area. My sister shoves a Coke and a piece of pound cake under my nose as I sit down at the table. "Whoa! How does anybody keep skinny around here?" I gasp as I gaze at the temptation in front of me.

"Oh, go ahead and eat. You can feel guilty later. Now, what's the latest gossip?" she says as she settles into the chair across from me.

Shaking my head, I grin at my sister and she grins back. And as I consume the scrumptious, empty calories before me, we talk of family and friends and husbands and jobs. And then, finally: "How's the treatment coming?" she asks. "Are you still? . . ."

I smile slowly and answer: "Yeah, we're still. . . . We're doing this last ditch sort of thing for another six or seven months at least."

"And then?"

I absently tap my plate with my fork. "Got any more of this fattening stuff?" I ask, moving toward the kitchen.

I cut myself a huge chunk and sit back down at the table.

"Lynda," my sister begins, then hesitates a moment. "What if you two never do have your own children?"

I stop in mid-chew as a flash of annoyance—no, stronger than that—anger rushes through me.

A young scream comes from another room. "I'll be right back," my sister says as she scurries toward the wail.

What if? . . . The words echo in my mind. I shove away from the table and walk out the back door and onto the redwood deck. *Crossing my arms, I lean up against a post.* Am I angry at my sister for asking the question? No, *I decide,* I'm angry at hearing it said out loud—out in the open, spoken words making it real, making it impossible to ignore.

"Well, all right then! What if *we* never?" I ask out loud. *The grass and the shrubbery give no reply. And as a gust of cool wind blows by, I hug myself tightly. Then as quickly as the anger came, it is gone.* Well, Lynda, *I think,* how **do** you feel about it all? *I squint, watching something move in a backyard several houses away. And then I hear the squeal of children playing.* Sometimes . . . I want a child so bad my insides literally ache with a longing that is real and whole and yet so—empty. But then, sometimes I look around me and see that things are all right, that children are nice, but that my life is still mine and that it can be full and meaningful with or without them. So. *I stop.* What *if* we never? . . .

"Hey, there you are. You okay?" *I hear my sister say from behind me as I hear the door slam and feel a hand on my arm.* "Look, I didn't mean to upset you. Really. I guess I just realize how much you do have, you know?" *my sister is saying.* "Like, your marriage, for starters. You two have a great one—any relationship that can get through what yours has is pretty solid, if you ask me. Having children is nice, but sometimes it isn't all it's cracked up to be. Believe me. Sometimes, I don't know, I . . ."

I turn to look at my sister. Another cry comes from the house— it's a mad cry. Tired, my sister rolls her eyes. "Benjamin has been stretching his terrible two's into another exciting year. He has really been a problem lately. I'll be right back."

I lean back against the post. How much I have. *Ten minutes ago, all I would have heard was a nice attempt to make me feel better by someone who cares for me. But, instead—this time—what I heard was . . . truth.*

I stride back into the house, pick up the phone and dial my home number. My husband answers.

"Hi, honey," I say.

"Well, hi. Is something wrong?"

"No, nothing's wrong. Just wanted to hear your voice."

"Lynda, you've only been gone four hours. Are you sure you're okay?"

I laugh, then sit down and prop my feet up on the phone table. "Yeah, I'm fine. Just fine."

SECTION 6

WHAT IF . . . NEVER?

The Resolution Crisis—
The Choices We Can Make

One weekend not long ago, I was reading the Sunday paper. It was filled with the usual amount of news, comics, helpful information. And as usual, I was doing an almost subconscious thing as I read. If I happened upon a useful piece of information that concerned baby care, pregnancy, or parental advice, I'd either clip it or mentally store it away for future reference. Maybe it was about a baby's need for dairy fat or how vitamin B6 helps curb morning sickness . . . This Sunday, it was a new device that works as a TV monitor with which you can actually keep an eye on your baby while doing other chores . . . I performed this little habit with other topics that affected my life. Why not this one? It never hurts to be prepared, you know.

But this Sunday's reading was different, because as I sat reading about this great new device, I let some repressed questions pop through: "Isn't this a waste of time?" "Aren't I going to be the most informed nonmother in the world?"

And then the corker:

"What if we . . . never have our own child?"

The part of me that's not ready to stop storing away helpful hints winced. But the rest of me, the realistic side of me that's beginning to rear its level head, realized I need to think about the possibility.

In my braver moments, I look the question straight in the eye, with chin out and arms folded: "Well, what *if* never?" Will I fall apart? Will I become a basket case, forever patting little boys and girls on the head? Or turn into one of those aunts that pinches cheeks? Or worse, will I spend the rest of my life recoiling at the sight of cute, cherubic-faced kids wherever they pop into view?

I suppose since I'm being honest about my fears, I should realize that the whole concept of asking "What if never?" is just that: questions, fears, apprehensions about the future— tensions. Yet as I put words to them, I also realize for the first time in this crisis that there are some choices I can make beyond whether to take this test or that treatment. When I decide to make them, when the time is right, there *are* choices I can make.

"Choices?" I can almost hear you shriek. "What do you mean choices! We've made the choice to have a child! I don't want to even *consider* a Plan B." Me, neither. The part of me that still mentally files away newspaper clippings hasn't let go. And as long as my husband and I are still attempting treatment, I will consider Plan B as still Plan B.

But I also know that unless Plan A comes through with that successful pregnancy, I *will* have to face Plan B. And one of the positive things about B, maybe the only positive thing, is that we can have control once more, even if we would never have chosen this sort of thing to control.

So, what if *never?*

There will come a moment in this crisis when your own realistic side will pop through with that question. You may be like us, dangling at the end of treatment that could go on indefinitely, or you may be part of this group yet have already thrown up your hands and said, "Enough!" You may have considered the technological answers, either exhausting them or deciding against them. Or you may have had the inescapable news of your absolute infertility thrust upon you, and the moment of realization came at lightning speed.

But for everyone who doesn't have a successful pregnancy, the moment will come. It is a moment that you *allow* yourself to think of Plan B, about the possibility, about the options, the choices, about redefining life as you want it to be.

Facing the "What if never?" question is not a demand for on-the-spot solutions. To ask it is to try the idea on for size, to get used to the idea that life goes on—and hopefully, to the idea that life does much more than just go on, that life can be *good* as it goes on. To think about "What if never?" is really a prelude to making a choice for the future, as scary as that sounds.

This type of choosing, though, is a gradual type—the same sort of timing you use to consider "What if never?" in the first place. It's a slow getting-used-to, working out of the tensions, the fears and apprehensions of each choice on the way to the one that's best for you as a couple. Doing it that way is healthy and is more likely to take you into the future more confident and at ease.

As a friend explained her and her husband's exploration of the adoption choice, it slowly showed them the limits and the avenues of the choice, and the limits and then the avenues of their own needs. Honestly and personally.

So what I feel we should explore in this last section is the crisis of choice at the end of the infertility quest—a close look at some of the tensions we may find ourselves grappling with before we can move confidently into the right choice for us. Hopefully, we'll be discovering, and then exploring, those limits and those avenues as we go.

Obviously, though, this can only be an informal look at the choices and their tensions. Detailed treatment of the specifics of adoption or childfree living are best covered in publications exclusively dealing with those topics. Our discussion is about the *unchanging tensions* that keep us from such study. So when you begin to explore these choices deeper, I'd encourage you to read everything you can get your hands on about either topic.

THE CHOICES

We've been talking about choices. Let's look at exactly what they are at this point:

- Stopping treatment and beginning adoption procedures.
- Beginning adoption procedures as you are going through infertility testing and treatment. Some adoption agencies will want you to stop infertility treatment and show signs that you've resolved your infertility when they call to say you're on their list. But until you hear such a request, you can choose to continue treatment. And because age is becoming a factor in adoption as well as fertility treatment, it may be the only feasible route for some.
- Stopping treatment and deciding to live "childfree."
- Proceeding with infertility treatment as long as you choose, but making your quest for a baby only one part of your life. Making goals, plans—going on with life as you continue treatment for now. Then, if a successful pregnancy happens, so much the better. If not, you'll have been building a meaningful life, and your future will not be *just* another anxiety you've put off.

"But how can I make such choices?" you may wonder. "I just don't have the emotional strength to handle anything like this now." Don't feel alone. The ongoing feeling of grief is a huge part of the infertility crisis, as we've discussed in Section 1, and especially of this stage of it. And grief takes all the fight right out of you, and all the straight-thinking judgment, too. But how we handle our feelings of grief is very much a part of asking, "What if never?" and still coming out the other end emotionally healthy, as we'll discuss later. So it's only normal for us to feel emotionally exhausted and hesitant to move on too quickly.

But here's the good news: There's no rush. You don't have to make any choice in the next thirty minutes, or even in the next month or year, especially as long as you feel emotionally and physically weary from grappling with infertility. In fact, the only thing worse for you to do beyond allowing the tensions of the choices to keep you from examining them is to jump into the choices too quickly. No one should push you into decisions until you are ready to make them. And *slowly* examining them—and yourself—is the best way to becoming ready.

But what if you can't *ever* make yourself look at any of the choices above?

Then, we should add another to the list above:

• Not making any choice at all.

You see, *not* making a choice is actually making one. And this is easy to do. It sort of sneaks up on you. How? Sometimes just simple inertia will keep you from facing the choices, or maybe the emotional trauma of infertility treatment is so awful that you cannot bring yourself to think about its long-term effects. And as time moves past, the choice is made for you.

The one truly dangerous thing about handling this end of the infertility crisis in such a way is that you not only allow the choice to make itself, you never make yourself face your feelings, your situation. Somewhat like your experience with infertility, you let it happen to you, feeling powerless, overwhelmed. Another verse of no control.

This can be a very natural reaction. Maybe without consciously realizing it, we don't believe we *can* take control of our lives. Isn't loss of control one of the major traumas of infertility? We may not believe control is even a possibility. We may be just too tired, too defeated to do anything in a positive sort of way. Yet, ignoring the problem does nothing for your wounded psyche, the part of you that makes for a healthy, productive future. So, not choosing *is* a choice, but far from an emotionally healthy one, for either of you.

Well, how do people finally choose?

There are as many ways toward these choices as there are people, I'm sure. Sometimes force of will—saying it's time to get on with life—will drive a couple to choosing one of the above. Sometimes force of biology in the shape of menopause is the first time many women will totally realize that "never" is here. The force of finances may have a hand in bringing treatment or adoption possibilities to a halt. For some, it's the force of ethics—when the new technology looks too "iffy." Sometimes even questionable forces motivate us, like hoping, as we've heard so often, that adopting will somehow help us have our own biological child. And then sometimes just the simple force of reality causes a couple to face the truth and carry on. But however the choices come to us, they come.

Still, the choices *are* ours when we're ready to make them. And after all we've been through, to have a choice, to take control once more is no small thing.

To get to those healthy choices, though, we need to jump some hurdles, emotionally and mentally, in as honest a fashion as possible. Let's begin by looking at the tensions of the first two choices, the ones concerning adoption.

CONSIDERING ADOPTION—THE TENSIONS

What are the tensions we feel as we first begin to consider adopting someone else's child?

Whether you begin to take steps toward adoption as you're still going through infertility treatment or whether it's after you've abandoned your quest for your own child, the tensions are much the same. Some of them are:

- You don't know what to expect. You've heard it is hard, almost impossible. Horror stories of years on waiting lists, of being turned down, of the scarcity of babies.
- You've heard the examinations and interviews are rigorous and personal, and you don't know if you're up to it.

- You may be worried because you and your spouse don't totally agree on adoption.
- You wonder if you'll have trouble accepting the child as your own.
- Your parents and friends are all asking you if you're going to adopt, some as if it's the solution, others as if it's not a good idea. And you're not quite sure how to feel.

ADOPTION PROCESS TODAY

True, adoption has changed drastically. Legalization of abortion, the widespread use of birth control, plus society's growing acceptance of young, unwed mothers keeping their babies have thrown the adoption situation into full reverse from what it was only a few years ago. And the results are all but catastrophic for those of us who choose to adopt. When we were growing up, adoption was looked on as a gesture of humanity. There were many more children than there were good homes to put them in. And the feeling that you were doing your part to help the sea of unwanted children was one of the good reasons for adopting. Now, in a strange way, it just may be more humanitarian of a couple *not* to adopt, so that another couple will have a chance . . .

Are babies really that scarce? Yes. Healthy white infants are. The only area where supply comes anywhere near demand is black infants available for adoption by blacks.[1] Laura Valenti, author of *The Fifteen Most Asked Questions about Adoption*, states that for every white healthy infant who becomes available for adoption, there are about fifty couples whose home studies are already completed and approved, anxiously waiting. Waiting lists are long and requirements are strict. In short, she says, "the competition is fierce."[2]

How do you go about adopting against such odds? In an article called "Adoption: It's Not Impossible," Andrew Wilson and Bradley Hitchings say that the first step is to overcome any shyness about it:

Going public means spreading the word that you want to adopt a child and getting in touch with those who have done it. You may need personal contacts and tips just to get you past the door at adoption agencies, and they're certainly vital if you decide to look into independent, noninstitutional arrangements.[3]

There *is* a group of children, though, that are not scarce for adoption: minority children, international children, and "Special needs" children (children who are older, children who need to be adopted with brothers and sisters, or who are handicapped mentally or physically). Much thought needs to go into *any* decision to adopt, of course. But even more realistic soul-searching should go into the adopting of these children. You'd need to ask yourself some in-depth questions, such as how important is it that the children be of the same race as you? How important is it to have an infant? Or do you have the emotional or financial resources to care for the special needs child? And those are just three of the things to ponder. It's emotionally healthy to realize our limits and accept them. And here is one of the specific places in adoption that doing so is crucial.

To begin the adoption procedure you'll need a list of the agencies in your state. You can get such a list from your state's Department of Social Services of Public Welfare. And the public library or the local public service adoption agency should be able to give you a list of private adoption agencies within the state. As rapidly as things change in American and foreign adoption, you should definitely research the latest books and magazine articles on the subject.

What should you expect after you begin contacting agencies? You'll find out how long each agency's waiting list is and decide if you want to be on it. A waiting list is a list of people who are waiting to be made active with the agency—"active" in the sense that they are part of the group that are "waiting," once again, to find out when they might adopt a baby. There are public adoption agencies, private agencies—many church-affiliated—that still maintain homes for unwed mothers, and there are some agencies that work only with special needs or international children. Some of the agencies have lists that are so long they are closed to new names; others are available only to people in a specific geographical area. Some agencies have age limits for the parents. And it is a safe assumption to say that as babies become even more scarce, the requirements will probably become more strict and more specific.

Private adoption, sometimes called "independent adoption," is another way to a baby, sometimes a much shorter one—but quite probably a more expensive one, since you'll likely be asked to foot all the pregnancy and birth expenses for things like rent, maternity clothes, food, and legal fees. Private adoption has become an alternative to agencies, but it *can* be laced with problems. Although laws attempt to keep it from turning into "black-market" adoption, there is still quite a bit of room for anything to happen. In several states private adoption is not even legal because of its inherent problems. And the newspapers have offered us enough stories about birth mothers backing out on such agreements to make us well aware of the tenuousness of this area of adoption.

One Los Angeles County Department of Adoption official reports that "there are countless cases in which couples pay a lawyer thousands of dollars for babies who turn out to be defective or haven't been carefully screened." And then he adds, "Some couples are so desperate for a child that they deal with the black market, the foreign market, the illegal market in babies. They pay all sorts of fees and in the end they get nothing but heartache."[4] As Wilson and Hitchings explain: "[C]aution is the watchword. Everything from faulty paperwork to outright scams is possible, and the consequences can be tragic."[5] Private adoption, hopefully undertaken with great care, is one alternative more and more couples are exploring, though, risks or no.

In short, yes, the adoption process can be very hard—and discouraging. And it may take years. But it's not impossible.

And I strongly urge you to come to terms with its difficulties in a positive way, not allowing yourself to look on the experience as an extension of your infertility "failures." It must be a deliberate, separate, much-studied choice, done open-eyed and open-hearted.

THE HOME STUDY

To discuss agencies, though, is to wonder how their requirements will affect us. The rigors, the scrutiny, the red tape of adoption agencies' studies—is it as bad as it sounds? How you respond to the interviews, questionnaires, and visits by social workers, what they call the "home study," may depend on how much you really want to adopt, why you want to adopt, and how well you've adjusted to your infertility. And that's a lot to think about. If you're worried about experiencing more hassle, you're probably not quite emotionally ready to adopt. But that's not to say you can't begin there. You can start the process toward adoption, and see how you respond. If you still find you're stuck and can't move beyond the past, you may not have worked through your raw feelings and into the place that you are ready to make such an all-encompassing decision. Adoption does not fit every couple's real needs. And though it may seem that every couple who can't have their own child ultimately adopts, it just isn't so. Not by a long shot. Too often we can feel pressured to adopt before we're ready to, and maybe when we really don't feel we want to.

Some people are able to come to that understanding alone. Others can only find out whether adoption is for them as they explore the choice deeper. If you're one of the latter, and you still find yourself apprehensive over the intrusion of the home study, think of it this way: Can anything be as bad as the intrusion that infertility has been to every fiber of our lives? Strangely enough, one friend who hesitantly began the adoption process found the adoption study's thoroughness to be a healing time:

I found there was a big difference between the part of my life when I languished in infertility testing, and the time I worked through the adoption study. Adoption was more humane, essentially. It was a time when I looked once again at myself as a whole person, after all those years of my fixation on just one part of me that wasn't whole and well.

Also, she feels the study was a time when she and her husband were pulled back together. Through the counseling sessions and the interviews, they were forced to talk about their feelings and to think about the future as a couple.

For so many years, our discussions were all centered around whose problem was causing this infertility. I've got this test; he's taking that treatment. Through the adoption work, we were looking at a new idea, not separately but together. It brought us back together by giving us common ground once again as a couple.

IF YOU DON'T AGREE

What if you and your spouse don't see eye to eye on the possibility of adoption? Now is the time to be deadly honest. We're talking about your lives and the future of a child. Now is *not* the time for worrying about feelings or for selfishly bull-dogging your wish through. It is a time to look at limits and avenues, just as we expressed it earlier. My friend quoted above wanted to adopt; her husband wasn't crazy about the idea. They agreed to begin the study, though, and she found her limits, he found some avenues. They were able to find common ground by voicing their real feelings. But it took counseling to get to that point, because they were so emotionally spent from the experience of infertility and so worried about what the choices might do to their marriage. For this couple, the home study helped them face each other and make a choice they both found comfortable.

Although the social worker who will be in charge of your home study may only seem to be a very powerful person who decides whether you get that baby or not, he or she is almost always a person who wants to match the child to the environment as perfectly as possible. Very realistically, though, the worker may look for signs that you're ready for this step, that you've worked through all such feelings, and have been open and honest with each other.

And that's a good thing, actually. In adoption, the issue is parenting. In infertility treatment, the issue is first and foremost pregnancy. The change in focus is what the adoption study can give you, and it may be exactly what you need to find out if adoption is the right choice for both of you.

SOCIAL PRESSURES

In reality, though, what *you* think is not the whole picture, is it? We know how very public our private decisions are when it comes to family-building. Why do strangers and coworkers and neighbors automatically ask you whether you are going to adopt? And while they're all taking it for granted you want to, why is Aunt Sally expressing concern over the possibility?

FAMILY

You may not want your family's opinion to matter much, but it does. And there's no getting around the tension involved with family feelings toward any new member to its ranks. If you're lucky, you'll have relatives who want what you want, no matter what you choose. But often, that's not the case, and you have to try to make your decision without the intrusion of their opinions. And that's hard.

Family members who are against adoption may be reacting to some personal attitude that could be open to change. Maybe it's some left-over feelings about adoption from another generation, maybe negative feelings about the family bloodline, maybe some prejudice about a foreign child. With a little effort, you may be quite surprised at their change in attitude if you take the time to talk with these family members.

But no matter what the situation, remember it is still your

decision, you and your spouse's. Just like the decisions you may have made about the new technological options, this decision affects you and your spouse and must be made by the two of you alone. Your lives are the ones truly affected. As we discussed in Section 2 on coping, these are times when you must try to understand the people around you by considering their spheres of reference, instead of allowing their comments to confuse or upset you.

OTHERS

Even if the family tension, the pressure from within, isn't so bad, the pressure from without—friends and others—is hard to ignore totally.

As I said before, social pressure is a crazy thing. We're already quite aware of its volatile nature through the infertility experience. When a stranger asks you if you're going to adopt, what is he or she really saying? Rarely is the person trying to persuade you to take this step. Why, then, do we get asked this so automatically? In a very real sense, adoption *is* seen by most people as a sort of "solution" for infertility. Yet, seeing adoption that way can cause all sorts of problems in our relationship with an adopted child. We can't go into adoption with that idea—and yet we still feel the pressure from around us and don't understand where it comes from.

ADOPTION AS THE SOLUTION TO INFERTILITY

"Can't have your own child? Well, don't worry, you can always adopt."

Why shouldn't we look at adoption as the "solution" for infertility? Because it isn't. The foremost problem with viewing adoption as a "cure" for infertility, or even as the next step in the infertility treatment, is that you don't have time to make peace with your infertility. And that, as we mentioned, may very well have far-reaching ramifications over how you relate to your adoptive child. Subconscious pressures that you would never consciously place on your new family might show up later.

What sort of pressures? Ones that may affect how you see the child and maybe how you accept the child. After eight long years of infertility treatment and finally adopting a son, one intuitive friend realizes the problem:

> I love my son very much. But adopting has not cured my problem. I'm still infertile. And to think of my son as a replacement for my own "dream child" would not only be unfair, but cruel. He'd have to live up to the image of my "perfect child" I couldn't have. No child should grow up under that tension.

Since society, contrary to reality or common sense, still may subtly suggest that adoption is the accepted substitute for having natural children, it must be said that the decision to adopt should never be made on such a basis. You owe it to the child you may adopt to keep him free of any negative loose ends still dangling from your infertility experience.

PARENTING VS. PREGNANCY—THE REAL ISSUE?

Yet, we still haven't considered *why* people automatically see adoption as the logical ending to an infertility experience. One possible answer is a concept that may speak volumes to our situation and toward our decision-making.

As mentioned before, adoption is really about parenting. Most people get the picture of our situation a little off-center. They think since we have gone to all the effort of infertility testing and treatment, we obviously want to parent. So, because they assume that parenting is what we want most, they naturally consider the next best way to parent is to adopt. On the other hand, whether we realize it or not, we may not have had parenting, per se, as our specific goal. Through all the infertility testing, our goal has been pregnancy. And that is where our focus may still be, and where much of our tension with the adoption choices may lie.

Barbara Menning, the founder of RESOLVE, sees the difference in the two needs, the two desires, quite plainly:

> [T]here are some people for whom the pregnancy and childbirth experience as well as genetic continuity are extremely important . . . and if this is denied them they don't want a child in any other way. Others find the parenting to be the larger thing. I was a maternity nurse, and, though I grieved at the sadness of not being able to make my own children, parenting was the overriding need for me.[6]

What's the difference between the two goals? A subtle one but a real one, I'm convinced. There may be some sort of built-in defense system that keeps us from grappling with the idea of our future parenthood until we're safely through the pregnancy—or nearly there. That's when the reality of what is happening comes through. It's probably the same way for most people, infertility or no. First, pregnancy is the goal. Then your future parenthood sinks in as you go through the process.

This idea is not something you may have thought about at all. And such a difference is not easily explained to an outsider. With a biological child, the feeling comes in a sort of natural, stepping-stone way, because the steps between being pregnant and becoming a parent follow so closely. With adoption, though, the reality of parenthood is thrust upon us suddenly. And that can cause quite a shock. Especially if we haven't settled in our minds the difference between the needs we were trying to meet with infertility treatment and the needs we are trying to meet with adoption.

The decision to adopt, then, is quite a different sort of decision from the decision to have a baby. Through infertility, we've been caught in the quest for pregnancy: Pregnancy, #1, Everything Else, #2. Adoption, on the other hand, is about the need to parent past that quest. And it is a whole different decision. Others may not understand that, naturally assuming that the goals are identical. Yet, as we begin to explore the avenue to the adoption choice, we can more readily see the reality, and the importance, of this difference. And then, understanding the difference, we can analyze our own limits to see if parenting is what we most want. Such self-examination may provide the deciding factor in our personal adoption question.

CHOOSING CHILDFREE LIVING—THE TENSIONS

A life without children. Obviously this is nowhere close to Plan A. Yet as you analyze the choices, you may want to know more about what a childfree life would be like. Why? There are several very good, very intelligent reasons.

1. Exploring the possibility of life without children can help calm any fears about what the future might hold. You might be worried about adoption not working out, maybe fearing in the midst of such strong emotion that childless living is unthinkable. But such panic can keep anyone from a clear-headed decision. And the intelligent couple will want to steer very clear of hasty decisions. Thus, as suggested in Section 2 on coping, you might want to ask yourself: *What is the worst thing that can happen? What is it about living without children that is so unacceptable?* Staring the possibility straight in the face can help you handle what does happen more effectively and sanely.

2. Examining the childfree choice can also be an exceptional way to clarify values and reevaluate *why* you want that child. You two have become different people on this end of the infertility struggle. It is easier to understand your attitudes about your real desire if you can explore exactly what bothers you the most about living without children. Then you'll be better able to analyze what your needs are now and how the choices can meet them.

3. Couples who have never felt comfortable with the idea of adoption, may want to know if life without children is livable. This also includes the situation in which you and

your spouse find yourselves at odds, leaning toward different choices. Together, you would be openly studying all the choices.

Make no mistake about it. The tensions surrounding the choices involving childfree living are very real and very tough—especially for the likes of us. Sometimes the apprehensions, the fears, the questions keeping us from a level-headed examination of this option aren't just hurdles. For some couples, those hurdles are so high they'll require a pole vault to get over.

But that's only natural. We've been focused so long on one goal—getting pregnant and having a child—that it seems ridiculous to think of not gaining that goal in some form.

"Having it all." That's the goal most of us had before infertility rearranged our plans. So many of us, thinking we could make all the choices, were shocked when we chose motherhood and didn't get it on schedule. Amazingly enough, I believe that many of us are still holding onto that mental attitude—tenaciously, if subconsciously. But very understandably. We just don't want to give up the idea that we can have it all. A dream is a dream after all. And dreams die hard.

One writer sums up our problem and its effects so very well. She says the infertile couple goes on, spending years and money

> . . . sometimes forgetting in the process why they wanted children in the first place, whether they'd make good parents, and what facets of their present childless life might be downright pleasant were it not for their focusing on what is missing.[7]

Ouch. That sounds too familiar. It hits where it hurts. Yet how else does a normal human being respond after spending a nice size hunk of one's life pursuing a dream? Still, the truth of that quote, and its telling assessment of the down side of our focused experience, is worthy of remembering as we trudge on.

REEVALUATING YOUR MOTIVES

Why do we want a child? Could it now be for some reason beyond wanting to parent? Could it be that the fortitude and determination which have gotten us through the infertility struggle have now pushed us into a tug-of-war with nature we're bound and determined to win?

What *does* a baby symbolize for you on this end of your fertility quest? *Now* is the time to ask.

It's too easy to get caught up in *the* quest, Holy Grail-style, and all but lose sight of the original feelings that you had. Think about it. Would you feel it irrational to choose not to have children after all the years of trying? It's easy to see such a choice as giving up, as being defeated. If so, then maybe your infertility struggle has become something bigger than just a quest for a child. One woman put it this way:

> I'm so caught up in trying to win the fertility battle that I don't even trust my own wish for a child anymore. It's become such an ego thing, such a power struggle, that I'm not even sure at this point why I'm doing it.[8]

Such an honest realization could be the beginning of a decision to remain childfree. As another woman who finally saw her own situation:

> . . . Being honest with myself, I can say that I've gotten caught up in an intense power struggle between myself and Mother Nature. At this point . . . the challenge of winning the power struggle has become more important than becoming a parent—although that's hard to admit! [But] once I give up the power struggle, I realize that I can be creative and productive without being PROcreative and REproductive.[9]

Think back to the pregnancy vs. parenting discussion under the adoption section. How did you feel as you ponder the difference between the two? What are your needs, your real "wants" on this end of the infertility road? What is spurring you on? You may come to realize that you are one of the large group of people who want a child of their own, but find that their limits stop this side of parenting for parenting sake. One man states the tensions this way: "Giving up the dream of pregnancy, bonding at birth . . . isn't easy, isn't always possible. No one should have to apologiize if they don't feel they can give it up in favor of adoption."[10]

As an echo of her explanation of the parenting vs. pregnancy needs stated earlier, Barbara Menning adds this thought:

> I think it's wise when people understand their needs and do not adopt if the childbirth and genetic considerations are that strong, because, then, an adopted child would be living reminder of their own infertility.[11]

Limits and avenues. Being honest with yourself about your real needs, at this point, can get you on the road to a decision. With such honesty, you can leave behind the pressure of what you, or others, think you *should* do in favor of doing what you need to do, or more importantly—what you need to *be*, no matter what you decide. You can have control again.

Well, okay, if we're talking honesty, what are some of the scenarios we envision for childfree living that have us worried?

- We wonder how it will be to break from the "normal" lifestyle we've grown up expecting, even if it isn't necessarily what's exclusively normal today.
- We wonder if we'll be going against the grain, and if we'll still be able to relate to friends who are knee-deep in childrearing.
- We wonder who'll take care of us when we're old.
- We wonder if we'll be sorry later.
- And we wonder if we'll be able to live without children in a society that continually reruns symbols of life achievements centered around family life—first day at school, graduation, wedding—like an old Kodak commercial.

Very easily, such fears can become motivations themselves.

And making a decision based on a fear or worry is asking for trouble later. So let's explore some of these tensions.

SOCIAL PRESSURES

If you look at such worries closely, you'll notice that they're almost all relational—social, how we relate to others and they to us.

MARRIAGE

The most special relationship you have is to your marriage. You want this relationship to be terrific. You started out dreaming that dream, and even though other dreams may have to be reshaped, this is one dream you want to be a reality on this side of the fertility battle. But what if you decide to live without children? Will it affect how happy your marriage will ultimately be?

I think you'd be surprised to learn how a significant number of people today feel about the connection between marital contentment and parenting. Angus Campbell, director of the Institute for Social Research at the University of Michigan, conducted a study on contentment in marriage and found that young married couples without children expressed the greatest contentment with their lives, followed by two groups: older couples without children, and older couples whose children were grown.[12]

Another study, done by the Roper Organization, states:

> Among the more significant findings is the overwhelming consensus that motherhood is no longer synonymous with marriage. While a majority of American women (94%) favor marriage, 82% do not feel that children are an essential ingredient for a happy marriage.[13]

Of course, there are also studies that show the flip side of the issue. And such differing studies just point to the problems of making blanket judgments on a topic like marital happiness in which there are as many factors involved as there are people and circumstances. But just the *fact* of such studies, virtually unheard of a generation ago, makes its own statement. Because however people assess their own childlessness or parenthood, there is no denying there's been a distinct change in attitudes regarding the element of parenting in marital and/or personal happiness. For example, when columnist Ann Landers asked her readers would they make the decision to parent again if they had the chance to do it over, a surprising majority responded negatively—70% of the fifty thousand that responded. Even taking into account that the question may have more readily pulled in those most disgruntled, the response is still strongly indicative of a change in social attitude.[14]

From the debate, though, there is at least one grain of truth for today. Marilyn Burgwyn, author of *Marriage without Children* says it well: "Marriage without children is not destined to be unhappy and unfulfilled any more than marriage with children is assured of being an unqualified success."[15]

Clarifying values. Reevaluating reasons and feelings. That's what these choices make you do. And it can be very good for your marriage. How you see yourself and your spouse, how you value each other will make a very telling difference in what your marriage might become without children. Your marriage may be one filled with the special vitality and closeness that sociologists have come to associate with many marriages without children.[16] But, marriage *is* what you make it, as one of my friends found out:

> When we finally realized we would never have children, I was worried how he would take it. I thought he would look at me differently, and look at us differently. But, instead, he said, "I married you for you." All these years of trying have changed us, I guess. We know now that we don't need kids to fulfill our marriage. We've got something more. I'm his best friend, and he's mine.

By now you have probably realized, as this couple has, that

placing your happiness around a child or anything besides each other is setting yourself up for hurt. "What if . . . never?" For your marriage, it all depends on what you make it. Communication, flexibility, total honesty—these are what are needed here, as you explore this choice. Then, if you choose to remain childfree, think of the time, the energy you have to spend on your marriage—the way you probably wished you could when you first married. A renurturing of those reasons you picked each other in the first place, and the dreams that went with them, can make all the difference.

OTHERS

Attitudes *are* changing. And a growing acceptance of marriage without children today lightens the social burden considerably for those who might choose childless living. Population expert Charles Westoff, head of Princeton University's Office of Population Research, has predicted that as many as twenty-five percent of women now in their twenties will not bear children.[17] That may sound less than amazing until we remember that not until this generation, just the last ten to twenty years, did women consider motherhood anything but a foregone conclusion. And by and large, this twenty-five percent are women who will *choose* from the beginning to live childfree—*without* going through the throes of infertility. Such a shift in social attitude has already opened doors for all women who ultimately remain childfree. We can already see the difference. Women now can find a myriad of places and ways to find fulfillment past the front door and the nursery. And being able to channel creativity and nurturing gifts in other ways in today's society makes a childfree life, however the choice was made, much easier to mold into something good.

But people are still people. And old attitudes formed in another generation can linger forever. One "You don't have any children?" delivered with a cocked eyebrow may do away with weeks of good, healthy coping. A lot of unfounded guilt floats around out there, waiting to clamp onto you, and you probably wonder where it's coming from and why—and more importantly, why you are susceptible to it.

Think back again to the parenting vs. pregnancy discussion under the adoption section. Just as people will casually misinterpret your need for adoption, they will also misunderstand your thoughts against adoption. An acquaintance sums up your situation, not understanding the dynamics of your struggle, and is surprised about your consideration of childless living. And then—worst of all—he or she *tells* you so, and the irrational guilt clamps on.

Once in a while, as I would attempt to answer someone's blunt query about adoption with an honest "I don't know," I've gotten indirect vibes that a less than gung-ho attitude about adoption was somehow selfish. Such an idea must be a hold-over from pre-abortion, pre-Pill days. In today's reality, altruistic concepts of adoption, although tinged with truth, don't totally apply anymore. As one psychologist expresses the situation: "[T]he truth is people do not adopt children to meet the needs of children. They adopt children to meet needs of their own."[18] And any of us at this stage of infertility can probably feel the truth in that statement deeply.

So the concept of being selfish or self-centered if one chooses to live without children is actually without any meaning at all. And the simple fact may be, in the words of one astute observer, that "it's far more common for selfish, immature people to have children for selfish, immature reasons."[19] As mentioned before, the most selfless gesture, sadly enough, may be made by the couple with ambivalent feelings toward adoption who decide to leave their spot in the waiting line to a couple whose need to parent is much deeper.

Still, social pressures are hard to ignore. Lynne Wood, who struggled with the idea of adoption before choosing to live without children, wisely sums up the pressure and our best response to it:

Having children is the American dream. Children are a part of a myth we go after whether it's the right thing for us or not. Even if you're infertile you still have choices to make. Those choices shouldn't be made to conform to cultural pressures.[20]

FAMILY

If you're the only hope for grandchildren, your parents may find it difficult to accept a choice for childfree living. If your aunts and uncles and cousins-once-removed place a big emphasis on the family name and on the importance of children, a decision to remain childless by you may generate some tired, old comments. But, again, it's your life, and even though old tribal attitudes are hard to break away from, you can still make your choice clear of any family tension—if you have to.

Just as with your infertility situation, though, honest communication with those you love, those you care for the most, is still the best avenue. Whether you get the support you need, the strokes you need at this crucial time can make quite a difference in how hard the tensions are to overcome. You might be surprised at your loved one's response, just as this woman was:

> When I shared the problem with [my mother-in-law] she said, "Honey, with all the problems raising kids, there's not much happiness in it. You'll probably live longer and have a happier life without them . . ."[21]

FRIENDS

We can't deny the fact. Many friends are rearing children. You've already noticed some alienation, probably, a natural drifting away between you. Will deciding to live childfree make the situation worse? Maybe, for a time. But very possibly, only for a time. We may underestimate the *power* of time to change things. Lynne Wood has seen it play a big part in her relationship with her friends who have children:

> It has become easier with time as children of friends grew older and I moved into my forties. In fact, I find now that as many of

my friends are dealing with the "empty nest" not only do I (and my husband, too) feel more in step with friends, but I also find myself supporting them through an experience not totally unlike my own.[22]

You may be pleasantly surprised to find that friends who are now consumed with parenting demands may in a few short years once again seek out your company.

Don't expect all your friends to understand, though. Especially other infertile couples. They, more than anyone, may fail to understand that choosing to live without children can be a positive step, even a success in your infertility struggle. Why would they not understand? They may see such a decision as threatening—because they haven't come as far as you have in the experience. They may still be denying their feelings about such choices, not ready to face them. Again, time *will* make a difference.[23]

REGRETS

What about regrets? Actually, who can get through any phase of life without them? Whether we have fifteen natural kids, seven adopted ones, or none at all, we all have days we wonder if we chose well, wonder what life would have been like "if. . . ." I've had enough friends who've either adopted or had children of their own tell me of such days to know that *everyone* wonders about life down "the road not taken." Of course, I have always done a terrific job of rationalizing my friends' problems away. You see, they had children; they didn't have room to gripe.

But one day, I was struck with what a difference perspective makes. A friend was telling me of her problems with her daughter, and I was listening sympathetically. But in the middle of it all, I thought—with the conviction cast from years of infertility: *She should be grateful for what she's got.* At that moment, she stopped, looked at me hard, and with the conviction cast from years of parental problems, said: "Lynda, you should be grateful for what you've got."

I almost laughed. I realized then, that the grass may always look greener, but it "ain't necessarily so."

In reality, any choice is a trade-off. There will be some good, some bad in any avenue we take. We probably know that deep-down. "I may not know a lot of the joys of motherhood," a woman expressed to me, "but I won't have a lot of the heart-ache either."

One writer interviewed both fertile and infertile couples who decided to live without children and asked them about their regrets:

> I was surprised to discover how well most people without chil-
> dren adjusted after they'd become "childfree." Even among those
> who had spent years battling infertility, I found few wholeheart-
> edly regretted not having children. Of course, the lives they lived
> were different than they might have been, but they came to see
> that difference as a fact of life—rather than a tragedy. The only
> people who regretted not having children were those who had
> not enriched their lives on their own, who had not used the extra
> time and resources that would otherwise have been spent raising
> children.[24]

Will you be sorry? Will you have regrets? Yes. Everybody does. But the cold truth is that you'll have regrets no matter *what* you choose. There will always be those moments of "what if. . . ." So, as Merle Bombardieri phrases it in her book *The Baby Decision*, a better question than "Will I regret my decision to remain childfree?" is "Which decision will I regret the least?"[25] Then, after choosing, we should all remember that any road we choose will have those days—rare ones hopefully—of second-guessing, and "what if-ing."

OLD AGE

We have an in-grained nostalgic portrait of old age in America—it's a cozy one with loving offspring gathered around us,
maybe at Christmas or Thanksgiving, all of them adoring us as

we swing on our country home's porch, a great-grandchild under each arm.

We know that such an image is out of some Norman Rockwell fantasy portrait, but many of us still believe it can be, and possibly should be. Is it any wonder, then, that we're concerned about what our later years will be like if we don't have children? *Do* we expect our children to take care of us? *Do* we think our happiness will depend on children and grandchildren?

I can't help contrasting the picture above with what one older lady told me. After asking about our situation, she said in a hushed voice: "Dear, don't you worry about it. Children turn sort of cockeyed when you get older. They either start wanting to make all your decisions for you or they ignore you all together. I've got four, so I know. They just become long-distance pains-in-the-neck. Be-lieeeeve me."

Oh, I believed her, all right. The truth, though, for most people, surely lies somewhere between the sweetness and light of the Norman Rockwell portrait and the tartness of the older lady's experience.

Interestingly enough, some recent studies on this very topic puncture big holes in our Rockwell portrait. One article from the *Journal of Gerontology* reports a study dealing with the wellbeing among older women without children. It found that, among married women, being childfree had no significant effects on how they felt about their lives. The results showed that what *was* "positively associated" with their attitude were their physical capacity, religious convictions, their quality of social interaction, and the strength of their social support.[26]

Another study, reported in *Family Relations Journal*, surveyed men and women ages seventy-two through ninety-six, some parents, some childless. Surprisingly, the study found that children did not assure less loneliness, more positive appraisals of life, or greater acceptance of death. So the study concluded that the "presence or absence of children does not appreciably alter the lives of the very aged."[27]

Maybe children aren't the hedge against loneliness and unhappiness we seem to envision them to be for later life. For one thing, what guarantee do we have that our children will live close enough to take care of us when we're old? In this mobile society, how could we ever be sure? Unless we were willing to pack our bags and follow them for the purpose of their taking care of us, we couldn't be sure.

A little realistic thinking will find the holes in this tension. Old age will be what *we* make it, and not what our kids make it. And in a very real sense, it would be unfair of us to cast our children in such a strings-attached role. No, we need to do our best to plan our own lives. As one RESOLVE member wrote: "We would make plans for providing for our old age, even if we *did* have a child."[28]

If we don't raise children, though, we might wonder if we will leave behind anything of value when we're gone. Such a fear is a legitimate one. We all want something we do to live on after us. But immortality doesn't come from having children. Even being remembered doesn't last too long. (One walk through a forgotten cemetery will prove that.) If wanting to make a difference in this world is important to you, making some lasting mark, think of all the careers that affect other people's lives—children's *and* adults'. You can easily throw your creativity and energy into a myriad of arenas that wil give you the feeling you're making that difference—here and now, with the people that are here and now.

Still, we may need to feel a sense of family, especially when our immediate family cannot give it to us for various reasons. Merle Bombardieri expresses this need and what we might do about it:

> We all need to feel connected to others, to know that there is more than one phone number to dial when we're depressed, more than one kitchen that's always open for tea and sympathy. This is one of the reasons why so many people mourn the loss of the old-fashioned extended family, all those aunts, uncles, and cousins living close by. Today, our high divorce rate and our penchant for mobility make it unlikely that many of us will have that

kind of extended family—at least one that's related to us by blood. . . . But we can form our own families. . . . Many couples feel that these "chosen" families meet their need for a sense of community better than our own blood relatives ever could . . .[29]

One of the best things about friendships is that they are the product of choice, not heredity. Merle is saying we can *make* extended family; we can choose them—and we can reap all the benefits from the choosing. "If you choose to remain childfree," she explains, "you are *not* relinquishing your potential for growth and intimacy. You will have two precious commodities—time and energy—to nurture already flourishing relationships and build new ones. . . ."[30]

Still confusing, isn't it? There are many, many more tensions I know you must be feeling. Making a list of them might help, applying the same honesty and openness to them as you have to the ones we've covered. Joining a support group, being around others who are considering the same sort of decisions you are, might be just what you need. And then maybe, at this point more than any other, you might consider getting counseling if you feel stuck. It's no secret that even the steadiest of marriages can falter over the tensions of such all-encompassing decision-making. It's truly up to you and your spouse to communicate, to work past these tensions, to honestly listen to each other's fears and apprehensions. Then, if you do find yourself stuck, it is more than smart to consider seeking outside help, whether you're stuck as a couple on the rightness of one decision over another, or whether you're pulling in separate directions.

GRIEF: RESOLUTION/ADAPTATION

No matter where you are right now in your decision-making, no matter what hurdle you're stretching to get over, you're probably wondering if you'll ever feel normal again. The answer to that may be in the way you handle your grief.

As discussed in Section 1, some people speak of "resolution"—a time of grief that is followed by a time when you feel sad but strangely buoyant, energy returned, spirits higher. Others speak of "adaptation," the concept of handling infertility and its griefwork like a chronic illness, with a series of changes, of periodic sadness and healthy readjustments.

I seem to be more in tune with adaptation. My feelings may be due to the nature of our own infertility—the type without a decisive end, with hope and possibility always dangling from it. With this sort of infertility, the hope finally turns into a brittle thing, and the possibility becomes something that haunts you instead of buoys you. It's the feeling that drives some couples to force resolution by purposely going through vasectomies or other sterilization procedures, or even using birth control again. For me, being able to adapt as I go, allowing for changes and adjustments, works well with my personal experience. Just to know it's okay to handle my grief in such a way is a big help. Grief as resolution seems to happen more with those who face "absolute infertility," who abruptly face their grief as they would a major loss, as in a death.

But allowing yourself to actually grieve over what you will never have is integral to moving forward in a positive way with life and with these choices, whatever form your grief takes. You grieving may be lonely since you most likely will be at a different point than your spouse, responding in different ways. And in reality, no one else may even know you are doing it. You may even find yourself grieving while you're still going through infertility treatment.

However the experience comes to you, whether your grief comes through resolution or adaptation, it's important to grieve for the child you may not have, for that dream you may not know, in order to break the deadly-fixed focus of infertility. Because whatever your ultimate choice at this point in your experience, it should be made after you've examined your own grief process. If not, your decision may be colored by how you feel, based on something besides your true needs.

It's a mistake, though, to think that any choice will alleviate all feelings of loss. Whether you adopt or not, the feelings are the same. You are grieving over the loss of potential, over a life picture. the grieving will take time to subside, and, if left unfaced, may never go away.

One couple after adopting two children still had overwhelmingly sad feelings when they thought about never having biological children. They felt guilty about the feelings for years, until, finally, they went to a support group and were able to air these feelings. There, they found such feelings were not unusual, and that even though they had chosen adoption, they were still "allowed" to grieve over their personal loss of never having their own biological child.

In a very real sense, I believe that we'll always feel a measure of pain. How can we not? The years of infertility are a part of our history. And just like any other pain in our lives, there's no big eraser in the sky that can smudge its marks off our lives, our psyches. Like other pain, it's a matter of living with it. One woman who's gone through all these emotions sees the tension this way:

> The only way to stop the occasional pain is to not be alive. Values can change; priorities can change. And they will change if we give them a chance to. But it doesn't mean we'll forget what we've been through.
>
> It's just that, one day, you make a choice toward positive living, and you just go on. And then it's like building a whole new landscape for your life. At first, it's a little barren, not much growing or blooming on it yet. But as you build, the landscape gets fuller and richer, and better and better—and better.

That's a good way of looking at our choices. We're beginning life anew. Rebuilding a life picture. A life landscape. And often, that means starting from scratch. But the landscape doesn't stay barren, if we don't choose for it to.

So can I grieve for a part of my life that may never be? I think so. But I believe that it will be almost impossible for me to come to this point without a change in attitude—and with the realization that I will now and then still feel the grief of my years of infertility—no matter what my choice.

But it will be up to me—to us—to take the focus off our infertility, and off children, and once again put it back where it was when we first married—on our relationship and our future.

We all can do that. First, we can allow ourselves to ask "What if never?" Then we all have the capacity to choose. And whether we believe it or not at this moment, we have the capacity to answer yes *and* no to all that goes with that rock-hard question. We have the capacity to say *yes*, we want to parent, or *no*, adoption is not for us. We have the capacity to say *yes*, I married you for you, and infertility doesn't change that. But most of all, we can say *no*, I will not allow this one part of our lives to take any more from our life together. And if we cannot make the choice for the future today, then we can tomorrow. Or the next day—because we're willing to face the tensions of the choices, mind clear and eyes open—taking control once again.

This is what I want for my husband and me. And what I hope for you, too.

EPILOGUE

"The only happy ending to an infertility story is a baby."

An article I recently read ended that way. And considering our "quest," there probably isn't one of us that wouldn't whole-heartedly agree.

But what really is a happy ending, anyway?

Is there only the kind that ends in baby bliss? And, for that matter, does a baby come with a guarantee of happily-ever-after? Of course, we know better. Guarantees don't come with any part of life, as we know all too well. So—what *is* a happy ending?

Well, I can only speak for myself, I suppose. My happy ending would include a baby. But whether the script includes one or not, I will still go for a happy ending.

I think my happy ending will be full of love and the quiet joy of living. In my happy ending, I will be valued, not because I'm somebody's mother or wife or daughter, but because I'm me. And because that's all I need to be. My happy ending will allow me first to be happy with myself so I then can be happy with all the others that tramp through my life, whether they be of my own making or not.

Can there be a happy ending to an infertility story without a baby? Beyond what I may feel now and then, I think the answer is a definite, hope-filled yes. Because the conviction I feel deepest is that our happy endings must come from ourselves if they are to come at all.

I wish for you a baby. But more than that—above everything—I wish for you a happy ending.

NOTES

Introduction

1. Matt Clark, et al., "Infertility: New Cures, New Hope," *Newsweek*, 6 Dec. 1982, 102.
2. Diane Harris, "What It Costs to Fight Infertility," *Money*, Dec. 1984, 202.
3. Diane Clapp, "DES: Its Impact on Infertility," RESOLVE medical fact sheet, 1983.
4. Roby Rowlands, "The childfree experience in the aging context: An investigation of the pro-natialist bias of life-span developmental literature," *Australian Psychologist* 17 (July 1982):141.

Section 1

1. Lori Andrews, *New Conceptions* (New York: St. Martin's Press, 1984), 97.
2. Barbara Menning, "Counseling Infertile Couples," *Contemporary OB/Gyn* (February 1979): 2.
3. Andrews, *New Conceptions*, 100.
4. Ibid.
5. Ibid, 101.
6. Patricia P. Mahlstedt, "The Psychological Component of Infertility," *Fertility and Sterility* 43 (March 1985): 335.
7. Deborah Larned Romano, "Looking for a Miracle," *McCall's*, February 1984, 28. Reprinted with permission from the February 1984 issue of *McCalls*.
8. Mahlstedt, "Psychological Component," 335.
9. Barbara Menning, "The Emotional Needs of Infertile Couples," *Fertility and Sterility* 34 (October 1980): 313.
10. Ibid.
11. Barbara Menning, *Infertility; A Guide for the Childless Couple* (Englewood Cliffs, N.J.: Prentice-Hall, 1977), 114.
12. Judith Stigger, *Coping with Infertility* (Minneapolis, MN: Augsburg, 1983), 23.
13. Ibid, 24.
14. Romano, "Looking," 28. Reprinted with permission from the February 1984 issue of *McCalls*.

15. Andrews, *New Conceptions*, 116.
16. Ibid, 112.
17. Romano, "Looking," 28. Reprinted with permission from the February 1984 issue of *McCalls*.
18. Stigger, *Coping*, 25.
19. Ibid, 84–85.
20. Menning, "Counseling," 2.
21. Mahlstedt, "Psychological Component," 340–41.
22. Menning, "Counseling," 2.
23. Stigger, *Coping*, 29.
24. Mahlstedt, "Psychological Component," 340.
25. R. B. White, H. K. David, and W. A. Cantrell, "Psychodynamics of depression: implications for treatment," in *Depression: Clinical, Biological and Psychological Perspectives*, ed. G. Usdin (New York, Brunner/Mazel, 1977), 308.
26. Mahlstedt, "Psychological Component," 337.
27. "Changing," RESOLVE National Newsletter, April 1985, 8.
28. Mahlstedt, "Psychological Component," 340.
29. Ibid, 339.
30. Menning, "Counseling," 4.

Section 2

1. Letter to the Editor, RESOLVE National Newsletter, April 1985, 7.
2. Mahlstedt, "Psychological Component," 335.
3. Lori Andrews, *New Conceptions*, 106.
4. Merle Bombardieri, "The Twenty-Minute Rule," RESOLVE National Newsletter, December 1983, 5.
5. Barbara Harvey and Allen Harvey, "How Couples Feel About Donor Insemination," *Contemporary OB/GYN* 9 (June 1977): 94.
6. Menning, *Infertility*, 120.
7. Andrews, *New Conceptions*, 117.
8. Ibid.
9. Menning, *Infertility*, 130.
10. Ibid, 153.
11. Andrews, *New Conceptions*, 115.
12. Menning, *Infertility*, 154.
13. "Empathy," RESOLVE National Newsletter, Dec. 1984, 1.
14. "Handling Those Comments," RESOLVE National Newsletter, September 1984, 3.
15. Maddison and Walker, "Factors Affecting the Outcome of Conjugal Bereavement," *British Journal of Psychiatry* 113 (1967): 1057.
16. Constance Shapiro, "The Impact of Infertility on the Marital Relationships," *Social Casework* 63, 7 (September 1982): 387–93.
17. "A Battle Won," RESOLVE National Newsletter, September 1984, 1.
18. Jeanne Fleming, Ph.D., "Infertility as a Chronic Illness," RESOLVE fact sheet.

19. Compiled from "The Stress of Infertility and How to Cope," RESOLVE National Newsletter, April 1981, 7; M Bombardieri, "Coping with the Stress of Infertility, RESOLVE fact sheet; and M. Bombardieri, "Coping with the Holiday Blues," RESOLVE fact sheet.

Section 3

1. Harris, "What It Costs," 202.
2. Stephen Corson, *Conquering Infertility* (Norwalk, CT: Appleton-Century-Crofts, 1983), 1.
3. Menning, *Infertility*, 4.
4. Ibid.
5. Rebecca Taylor, "Understanding Fertility Problems," American Fertility Society booklet, (Daly City, CA: Krames Comm., 1983), 3.
6. Sherman Silber, *How to Get Pregnant*, (New York: Warner Books, 1980), 56.
7. Ibid, 57.
8. Ibid, 59–60.
9. Joseph Bellina, M.D., Ph.D. and Josleen Wilson, *You Can Have a Baby*, (New York: Crown Publishers, 1985), 86.
10. Menning, *Infertility*, 17.
11. B. Schwartz, R. W. Rebar, and S. S. C. Yen, "Amenorrhea and long distance running," *Fertility and Sterility* 34 (1980): 306.
12. Corson, *Conquering Infertility*, 35.
13. Mary Harrison, *Infertility: A Guide for Couples* (Boston: Houghton-Mifflin, 1979), 33.
14. Menning, *Infertility*, 18–19.
15. Corson, *Conquering Infertility*, 34.
16. Silber, *How to Get Pregnant*, 2.
17. Menning, *Infertility*, 19.
18. Ibid, 19–20.
19. Ibid, 24.
20. Harris, "What It Costs," 202.
21. Ibid, 206.
22. Taylor, "Understanding Fertility Problems," 3.
23. Diane Clapp, "An Overview of the Infertility Work-up and the Tests Used," RESOLVE medical fact sheet, 1984.
24. Harris, "What It Costs," 208.
25. Corson, *Conquering Infertility*, 48.
26. Clapp, "Overview of Work-Up," RESOLVE fact sheet.
27. "Semen Analysis," RESOLVE medical fact sheet, 1980.
28. Corson, *Conquering Infertility*, 54.
29. Ibid.
30. Harris, "What It Costs," 206.
31. Diane Clapp, "Medical Updates," RESOLVE National Newsletter, June 1985, 7.
32. Corson, *Conquering Infertility*, 54.
33. "H.M.G. (Pergonal)," RESOLVE medical fact sheet, 1980.

34. M. Schwartz and R. Jewelwicz, "The Use of Gonadotropins For Induction of Ovulation," *Fertility and Sterility* 35 (January 1981): 10.
35. Clapp, "Overview of Work-Up," RESOLVE fact sheet.
36. Dr. Robert Hunt, "Hysterosalpingograms: Facts You Should Know," RESOLVE National Newsletter, December 1981.
37. Clapp, "Overview of Work-Up," RESOLVE fact sheet.
38. Corson, *Conquering Infertility*, 60–61.
39. Claudia Wallis, "The Career Woman's Disease?" *TIME*, 28 April 1986, 62.
40. Corson, *Conquering Infertility*, 137–41.
41. "Immunologic Infertility," RESOLVE medical fact sheet, 1980.
42. Dr. Hugh Melnick, "Sperm Processing and Intrauterine Insemination," RESOLVE National Newsletter, April 1984.
43. Diane Clapp, "Artificial Insemination by Husband or Donor Sperm," RESOLVE medical fact sheet, 1983.
44. Earl Ubell, "Encouraging News for Childless Couples," *Parade*, 6 May 1984, 11–13.
45. Lois Goulder, "The Dilemma of Concealed Conception," *Family Weekly*, 26 May 1985, 8.
46. Nancy J. Alexander et al., "Artifical Insemination," booklet (Portland, OR: The Oregon Health Sciences University, 1984), 16; Corson, *Conquering Infertility*, 148–49.
47. Alexander et al., AI booklet, 5.
48. Silber, *How to Get Pregnant*, 179.
49. Lane Lenard, "Hi-Tech Babies," *Science Digest*, August 1981, 86.
50. "Third Frozen Embryo Birth Filmed," *Dallas Morning News*, 18 Aug. 1984.
51. "Troubling Test-tube Legacy," *Newsweek*, 2 July 1984, 54.
52. Silber, *How to Get Pregnant*, 187.
53. Diane Clapp, "In Vitro Fertilization: An Overview," RESOLVE medical fact sheet, 1984.
54. Ibid.
55. Maleia Olson and Nancy Alexander, "In Vitro Fertilization and Embryo Transfer," booklet (Portland, OR: The Oregon Health Sciences University, 1984): 39.
56. Glenna Whitley, "The Baby Race," *Dallas Life* (*Dallas Morning News Magazine*), 28 April 1985, 11.
57. S. Siwolop, "In Vitro Fertilization Isn't the Stork of the 80's," *Business Week*, 3 March 1986, 88–89.
58. Olson and Alexander, I.V.F. booklet, 35.
59. Joan Liebmann-Smith, "In Vitro Fertilization: What You Might Not Be Told," *American Health*, November 1985, 79; Meg Phillips, "One Woman's Courage," *American Health*, November 1985, 76.
60. Siwolop, "I.V.F. Isn't the Stork," 89.
61. Clapp, "I.V.F. Overview," RESOLVE fact sheet.
62. "Maryland Insurance Must Cover In Vitro," RESOLVE Newsletter, June 1985, 1.
63. Olson and Alexander, I.V.F. booklet, 37–38.
64. Andrews, *New Conceptions*, 151.
65. Olson and Alexander, I.V.F. booklet, 1.
66. Diane Clapp, "Medical Updates," RESOLVE National Newsletter, June 1985, 6.

67. "Surrogate Mother Programs," RESOLVE medical fact sheet, 1984.
68. Dame Mary Warnock, et al., *Report of the Committee of Inquiry into Human Fertilisation and Embryology*, (London: Her Majesty's Stationary Office (HMSO), July 1984): 47.
69. "Surrogate Mother Programs," RESOLVE fact sheet.

Section 4

1. Bruce L. Anderson, *The Price of a Perfect Baby* (Minneapolis, MN: Bethany House, 1984), 17.
2. Warnock et al., *Report of the Committee*, 6.
3. Lori B. Andrews, "Yours, Mine and Theirs," *Psychology Today*, Dec. 1984, 20–29.
4. Joan C. Amatniek, "Conference Examines the Scientific Status of New Reproductive Technologies," *OB/Gyn World* 2 (April 1985): 19.
5. Harvey and Harvey, "How Couples Feel," 93.
6. Andrews, *New Conceptions*, 276.
7. Andrews, "Yours, Mine and Theirs," 21–24.
8. Ibid.
9. Ibid.
10. Ibid.
11. Ibid.
12. Andrews, *New Conceptions*, 171.
13. George J. Annas, "Artificial Insemination: Beyond the Best Interests of the Donor," *Hastings Center Report* 9 August 1979): 14–15, 43.
14. Warnock et al., *British I.V.F. Report*, 27.
15. Andrews, *New Conceptions*, 169.
16. Ibid, 172.
17. Ibid, 169.
18. Andrews, "Yours, Mine and Theirs," 27.
19. Ibid, 28.
20. Ibid, 29.
21. Ibid.
22. Andrews, *New Conceptions*, 188.
23. D. Gareth Jones, *Brave New People* (Grand Rapids, MI: Wm. B. Eerdmans Publishers, 1984), 129.
24. "Views on A.I.D.," RESOLVE medical fact sheet, 1984.
25. Henlee Barnette, *Exploring Medical Ethics* (Macon, GA: Mercer University Press, 1982), 84.
26. Marion Duckworth, "Artificial Family," *Solo* 1, ed. 40 (1985): 28.
27. D. Gareth Jones, *Brave New People*, 128.
28. Ibid.
29. Andrews, *New Conceptions*, 148.
30. Ibid.
31. Richard J. McCormick, "Ethical Questions: A Look at the Issues," *Contemporary OB/GYN* 20 (November 1982): 227–38.
32. Howard W. Jones, Jr., "The Ethics of In Vitro Fertilization—1982," *Fertility and Sterility* 37 (February 1982): 147.

33. "Test-Tube Legacy," *Newsweek*, 54.
34. Jones, "The Ethics," 147.
35. D. Gareth Jones, *Brave New People*, 168–69.
36. Leroy Walters, "Human In Vitro Fertilization: A Review of the Ethical Literature," *The Hastings Center Report* 9 (August 1979): 25.
37. McCormick, "A Look at the Issues," 227.
38. Colin Honey, "The Ethics of In Vitro Fertilization and Embryo Transfer," *Modern Churchman* 26 (1984): 3.
39. Clifford Grobstein, "The Moral Uses of 'Spare' Embryos," *The Hastings Center Report* 12 (June 1982): 5.
40. Honey, "The Ethics," 3.
41. Leon Kass, "Making babies—the new biology and the 'old' morality," *Public Interest* 26 (1972): 18, 56.
42. Martin Mawyer, "So What's Wrong With Test-Tube Babies?" *Moody Monthly*, September 1982, 129.
43. Clifford Grobstein, Michael Flower, and John Mendeloff, "External Human Fertilization: An Evaluation of Policy," *Science*, 14 Oct. 1983, 127.
44. Grobstein, "Moral Uses," 5.
45. Amatniek, "Conference on New Reproductive Technologies," 21.
46. Whitley, "The Baby Race," 10.
47. Warnock et al., *British I.V.F. Report*.
48. "Test-tube Legacy," *Newsweek*, 54.
49. Amatniek, "Conference on New Reproductive Technologies," 21.
50. Whitley, "The Baby Race," 10.
51. Honey, "The Ethics," 3.
52. Paul Ramsey, "Shall We Reproduce? II. Rejoinders and Future Forecast," *Journal of the American Medical Association* 220 (5 June 1972): 1481.
53. Allen Verhey and Lewis Smedes, "Test-tube babies," *Reformed Journal* (September 1978): 17.
54. "Test-Tube Legacy," *Newsweek*, 54.
55. "France: Love In a Legal No Man's Land," *Newsweek*, 16 July 1984, 44.
56. Grobstein et al., "External Human Fertilization," 129.
57. Repository for Germinal Choice," *New York Times*, 14 July, 1982.
58. Robert H. Blank, "Making Babies," *The Futurist*, Feb. 1985, 15–16; Robert G. Wells, "The Hidden Costs of the New Genetics," *Moody Monthly*, June 1984, 70.
59. Blank, "Making Babies," 16.
60. "Human Life and the New Genetics," A Report of Task Force Commissioned by National Council of Churches of Christ in USA, (New York: Office of Family Ministries and Human Sexuality, 1980): 18.
61. Lenard, "Hi-Tech Babies," 86.
62. Andrews, *New Conceptions*, 224.
63. Janet Dickey McDowell, "Ethical Implications of In Vitro Fertilization," *Christian Century* 19 (October 1983): 938–39.
64. Kenneth B. Jones, "Surrogate Motherhood and Criminal Law," *Pennsylvania Medicine*, January 1984, 22.
65. Quoted in Beverly Freeman, "Facing the Ethical Issues," RESOLVE National Newsletter, June 1983, 1.
66. Angela R. Holder, "Surrogate Motherhood: Babies for Fun and Profit," *Law, Medicine, and Health Care* 5 (June 1984): 115.

67. Corson, *Conquering Infertility*, 151; Whitley, "The Baby Race," 36; "Can Science Pick a Child's Sex?" *Time*, 27 Aug. 1984, 59.
68. Whitley, "The Baby Race," 30.
69. Susan Lang, "Conceivable Sex Selection," *American Health*, May 1986, 10.
70. "Predetermining A Baby's Gender," *Parade*, 20 July 1986, 8.
71. Alvin Toffler, *Future Shock* (New York: Random House, 1970), 204.

Section 5

1. Verney and Smedes, "Test-tube," 18.
2. Lewis Smedes, *Forgive and Forget* (San Francisco: Harper & Row, Publishers, 1984), 91.
3. "Letter to the Editor," RESOLVE National Newsletter, June 1985, 4.
4. C. S. Lewis, *The Problem of Pain* (New York: MacMillan & Company, 1962), 39.
5. Bruce Shelley, *Christian Theology in Plain Language* (Waco, TX: Word, Inc., 1985), 97.
6. Philip Yancey, *Where Is God When It Hurts* (Grand Rapids, MI: Zondervan, 1977), 57.
7. Ibid, 67, 77.
8. James Dobson, "The Childless Couple," *To Be a Woman* cassette album (Waco, TX: Word, Inc., 1983).
9. Mari Haynes, *Beyond Heartache* (Wheaton, IL: Tyndale House, 1984), 88.
10. Yancey, *Where Is God*, 73.
11. Ibid, 88.
12. Evelyn Underhill, *The Spiritual Life* (Wilton, CT: Morehouse-Barlow Publishing Co., 1955), 20.

Section 6

1. Andrew B. Wilson and Brandley Hitchings, "Adoption: It's Not Impossible," *Business Week*, 8 July 1985, 112–13.
2. Laura Valenti, *The Fifteen Most Asked Questions about Adoption* (Scottsdale, PA: Herald Press, 1985), 35.
3. Wilson and Hitchings, "Adoption," 112.
4. "Babies Wanted," *Parade*, 30 Sept. 1984, 19.
5. Wilson and Hitchings, "Adoption," 112.
6. Diana Burgwyn, *Marriage without Children* (New York: Harper & Row, Publishers, 1981), 105.
7. Ibid, 94.
8. Merle Bombardieri, "Childfree Decision-Making," RESOLVE fact sheet.
9. Ibid.
10. Ibid.
11. Burgwyn, *Marriage Without Children*," 105.
12. Ibid, 16–17.

13. "Research Shows Childfree Marriages Happiest," National Alliance for Optional Parenthood (NAOP) Newsletter, January–February 1975.
14. Marian Faux, *Childless by Choice* (Garden City, NY: Anchor Press, 1984), 2.
15. Burgwyn, *Marriage Without Children*, 105.
16. Faux, *Childless by Choice*, 5.
17. Ibid, vii.
18. Margaret McDonald Lawrence, Conference Presentation, "Inside, Looking Out of Adoption," American Psychological Association, Washington, D.C., September 1976.
19. "Childfree Decision–Making," RESOLVE fact sheet.
20. Ibid.
21. Burgwyn, *Marriage Without Children*, 101.
22. "Childfree Decision–Making," RESOLVE fact sheet.
23. Ibid.
24. Ibid.
25. Merle Bombardieri, *The Baby Decision* (New York: Wade Publishers, Inc., 1981), 47.
26. Linda J. Beckman, "The consequences of childlessness on the social–psychological well-being of older women," *Journal of Gerontology* 37, 2 (March 1982): 243–50.
27. Pat M. Keith, "A comparison of the resources of parents and childless men and women in very old age," *Family Relations: Journal of Applied Family and Child Studies* 32, 3 (July 1983): 403–09.
28. "Childfree Decision-Making," RESOLVE fact sheet.
29. Bombardieri, *The Baby Decision*, 135.
30. Ibid, 134.

APPENDIX

RESOLVE, Inc.
P.O. Box 474
Belmont, MA 02178-0474

Founded in 1973 by Barbara Menning, a nurse going through infertility herself, RESOLVE is a national self-help infertility organization in existence essentially to help those facing infertility. With its telephone hotline, its referral service, its clearinghouse for medical information, and its support group chapters across the country, RESOLVE provides a service that every couple facing the trauma of infertility can benefit from in one form or another. Its national headquarters offers telephone counseling, medical consultation, an information-packed newsletter, and continual counseling helps and medical updates in the form of fact sheets available for public purchase. (The national office fields 50,000 literature requests and 250,000 information requests annually from members and the general public.)

Recently RESOLVE has also undertaken advocacy efforts, working to shape public opinion on issues affecting infertile couples, such as allocation of funds for research and broader insurance coverage. The organization is supported by RESOLVE memberships and sales of its literature.

For more information, call (617) 484-2424, or write to the address above.

American Fertility Society
1608 13th Avenue South, Suite 101
Birmingham, AL 35256-6199

American Fertility Society is the national professional organization for fertility specialists. It provides referrals to physicians, but also publishes literature that can help us understand the medical side of infertility better, as well as the medical journal *Fertility and Sterility*. Write to the above address for more information on pamphlets and referrals it might be able to provide.

INDEX

242